while you're down there...

while you're down there...

how to ask for what you want in bed – and get it!

Emma Dickens

Michael O'Mara Books Limited

First published in 2006 by
Michael O'Mara Books Limited
9 Lion Yard
Tremadoc Road
London SW4 7NQ

Copyright © Michael O'Mara Books Limited 2006

Michael O'Mara Books Limited disclaims any liability for anything
that may occur as a result of information given in this book.

All rights reserved. No part of this publication may be reproduced,
stored in a retrieval system, or transmitted by any means, without
the prior permission in writing of the publisher, nor be otherwise
circulated in any form of binding or cover other than that in
which it is published and without a similar condition including this
condition being imposed on the subsequent purchaser.

A CIP catalogue record for this book is available from
the British Library.

ISBN (10 digit): 1-84317-199-6
ISBN (13 digit): 978-1-84317-199-7

1 3 5 7 9 10 8 6 4 2

Designed and typeset by E-Type

Printed and bound in Great Britain by
Cox & Wyman, Reading, Berks

www.mombooks.com

contents

Author's Acknowledgements	7
Foreword	9
Chapter One: Here's Looking at You	12
Chapter Two: The Art of Communication	35
Chapter Three: The Sex Factor	56
Chapter Four: Let's Get It On	77
Chapter Five: Sexual Troubleshooting	104
Chapter Six: Spice Up Your Sex Life	123
Conclusion	153
Appendix: Back Passages	155
Bibliography	158
Index	160

author's acknowledgements

My thanks – and congratulations – to anyone who reads this and recognizes themselves, despite my attempts to disguise them. Thanks also to Victoria Alers-Hankey, Lindsay Davies, Kate Gribble, Candida Royalle, Kate Taylor and, most of all, to my Nick.

foreword

The writing of this book has introduced me to a surprising phenomenon. When I tell women what I'm writing and that it is to help women tell men what they'd like in bed, their eyebrows shoot up. They don't shoot up in a 'ooh-sex-how-risqué' way or a 'poor-women-who-need-a-book-like-that' way. It is an unmistakeable expression: it says, 'Imagine such a book. That's what I need.'

ABOUT THIS BOOK

I once met an old man on a train who had been married five times. He said that in a partnership, sex, when it was right, was about 5 per cent of the relationship; whereas when it was wrong, it was about 90 per cent. For most of us, though, the problem is not as monumental as that; it's more of a niggle. Perhaps you've got out of the habit of sex or you're in a rut with it. After a while, you and your partner need to learn to see each other as sex objects again.

Sex guru Kate Taylor, author and former sex expert for *The Sun* and *GQ* magazine, thinks we're all in a fix because of her White Knight theory of sex: we think that when we meet the 'right' man, the sex will be fantastic;

he'll just know what our body needs to feel alive and the simple touch of our lips on his will make him swoon with ecstasy. 'No, no, no,' Taylor says. 'This is sweet, but it's not true. It's like saying, "When I meet the right car, I'll know how to drive."' How right she is. Sex isn't automatically successful. It demands patience and a lot of practice. This should be easy to achieve, but in reality partners sometimes need to remind each other to have sex at all.

We need to blaze a trail for women ... and sulk until he asks us what's wrong. Not really: we must *act*. Unlike other sex books, knowing that words and time are both precious, *While You're Down There ...* will not waste either describing the missionary position to you. This is a targeted book. If, on the other hand, something is perhaps unfamiliar – Coital Alignment Technique or kegel exercises for men, maybe – I will talk you through it to clarify, unlocking the secrets of the so-called 'sexperts'.

A great sex life is not based solely on knowing tricks to enliven your lovemaking, though – it's also about being well matched outside of the bedroom. Accordingly, contained herein are some sure-fire relationship tips, to ensure that you're communicating with your partner on an emotional as well as a physical level. If you can't talk to each other about the day-to-day, sooner or later the talking dirty will dry up – that's a fact.

Speaking of which, *While You're Down There ...* will unpick the facts from the fiction. Sex clichés abound. Though some are well founded – women like lots of foreplay, men are stimulated by pictures, for example – others need refining. The idea that women are emotional about sex, for one. We are, certainly, but not all the time – and of course men have a range of responses beyond 'she has pulse: must fuck' too. This book will explode those assumptions that can be damaging to a sexual relationship, as well as pointing you in the right direction for a sex life that will be both stimulating and satisfying.

The volume is structured in a distinctly female way: first set your own lands in order, it says; then learn to talk to your partner; then start paying attention to the sex itself. Once you've got the basics down pat, begin to throw in some extras to take things to a more adventurous place.

Let's get it on.

chapter one
here's looking at you

Generally contented as you are, ever feel like you're not quite getting the hot sex you deserve?

Before we lay the blame squarely on men's shoulders, we must first focus on ourselves. Not necessarily because we're the root cause of the problem (a particularly – and, ironically, often damagingly – female approach, always to attribute culpability to ourselves), but because understanding and appreciating our own sexuality is one small step for us, one giant leap towards the sensual sex of your dreams. Think about this: if you know what turns you on, you'll be well equipped to share that knowledge with a lover. But if you're both in the dark, all that fumbling has no focus.

As far back as women can remember, we've been putting others first. But if we fail to recognize that we have needs as well, we are at least partially responsible for some of our problems. If you don't keep track of your sexual needs and satisfy them, you'll end up resentful and disappointed. You've heard it a thousand times before, but you've ignored it: you must learn to love yourself if others are to love you too.

DID YOU KNOW?

Fifty-one per cent of women prefer sex with the lights off, compared to 27 per cent of men. In a 2001 survey by *Top Santé* magazine, out of 3,000 women – average age thirty-eight – 95 per cent said the appearance of their bodies depressed them; 42 per cent preferred to undress with the lights off; two thirds said they would have better sex if they had an ideal body. Uh oh.

LET'S GET YOU READY, LADY

Before we begin dishing out advice to him, let's focus solely on you. This book has probably come into your possession because the Garden of Love, while beautiful, could do with a little maintenance.

First things first: forget the fairy tales. A survey conducted in 2005 suggested that those brought up on fairy tales were less likely to be capable of holding down a relationship. This might be news to you, but the key to a lifetime of romance is not to collapse into your man's arms and let him take you over. Not all the time, anyway. You need to be assertive in a relationship – it's the only way for both of you to maintain that spark.

The secret to enjoying anything is to participate in it as fully as you can. Your man could train for hours in the art of cunnilingus, taking in all the information and tips in the world, but unless he senses that you're with him all the way, your relationship isn't the two-way street it needs to be in order for it to be rewarding for both of you. You need to take control of your own sexuality and both of you need to be willing and able to take direction from the other. Think of yourselves as sexual pioneers, embarking together on a voyage of discovery.

14 \ while you're down there ...

In order to take charge of your own sexuality, you need to find out as much about yourself and your desires as you can. Encourage him to do the same, eventually, but we're focusing on you for the moment.

If I Could Choose Anything ...

Get yourself into the groove of self-discovery by trying the following exercise. In the first instance, work your way through the steps alone. Of course, this also works well with a partner, and you may want to share the process with him later, when hopefully it will mark the beginning of a rich fantasy life between you. Just for the moment, though, it's all about self, self, self.

1 Set aside half an hour or an hour.
2 Resolve not to answer the phone or the door.
3 Get yourself comfortable, perhaps on your bed or on the sofa.
4 Close your eyes.

Now for the fun part:

1 Become aware of your body and let your mind wander sexwards.
2 Start to contemplate sexy scenarios, taking your time as you do so.
3 Now visualize your ideal sexual experience and let it run its course from beginning to end. Savour it.

How was it for you? Think back over your favourite fantasy:

- Where were you?
- Who, if anyone, were you with?

- What engaged your senses? Particular aromas? Food? Drink? Silk? Fur? Sand?
- Was it a long, languid experience or a sudden, spontaneous one?

What did you learn? Any surprises? Did you masturbate? Bet you will next time, if you didn't this. This is your fantasy, so now do with it what you will. For the moment, you might want just to remember it when you're on your own again. Or do you want to share part or all of it with your partner? Do you want to keep your gloriously sordid inner life a secret? Or on the contrary do you want to act it out?

Did you know?
Six out of ten people have had sexual fantasies that they didn't share with their partners.

Dream a Little Dream

If you're in need of inspiration, or permission to unlock your imagination, here are some of the things that have featured in bona fide women's fantasies. They're fairly racy, as you might expect. Women's sexuality unleashed is not a demure little thing wrapped up in gingham with a pretty pink bow. It's often filthy, hard-core, give-it-to-me-now, demanding, rampant, wonderful stuff. Don't get me wrong: the slow, sensual approach – candles, massages, making sweet love with the man of your dreams – has its place in a woman's sex life. But the fantasies that tip us over the edge are not often packaged up with fairy-tale trimmings. Forget any preconceptions

16 \ while you're down there ...

you may have about your sexuality and your desires right now. Be open about going beyond any boundaries in your mind. Remember these are only fantasies – unless you want to make them real. There's every difference between thinking something and acting on it. Don't be scared. Dare to daydream.

WOMEN'S SEXUAL FANTASIES

Gang bang: featuring husband's suited colleagues

With your best friend in a sauna

Champagne in wide champagne glasses – for dipping your breasts into, of course

Four men: one in your mouth, one inside you and one in each hand

Prim schoolmistress with no knickers on, with a slow male pupil

Being taken from behind by a stranger at a football match (while the crowd's distracted by the excitement of the game)

Having a penis and fucking your partner

Strip poker with a stranger

Your best friend, who's fucking your boyfriend, who tries to resist – but is overwhelmed by desire

A motorcycle courier, who orders you to tell him what you want or he'll take you anyway

Getting caught masturbating by a neighbour

Several women at once going down on you in a women's prison

Being seventeen and getting caned by the headmistress, among other teachers

Starring in a sexy photo shoot, which evolves into a full-on sex session, all caught on camera

here's looking at you / 17

Playing sardines, being found by your favourite playmate, fucking when you're about to be found by the others

A carrot inserted in your arse

Being taken by a priest in the confessional box after confession

Being taken against your will

A woman with large breasts pushing a cold bottle up inside you

Having the boss's cock in your mouth and being watched by the rest of the office, who are all thoroughly aroused

Getting paid for sexual acts by a john

Being taken by someone who picked you up hitch-hiking

Your neighbour watching you in your bathroom through a secret hole, which he's been doing for years. He found out about it from the neighbour before and so on

Having a hose stuck inside you

Being back at school and being taken by a boy who's a pupil there, while your brothers look on, instructing him

Your mother, who's showing your body off bit by bit to a rajah

Being put through your paces in bed by a famous pop star

Gang bang: you in a mask with a queue of men you never see

A faceless woman playing with and sucking your breasts, while you masturbate

Appearing in a hard-core porn film, and imagining the effect you're having on all the viewers

Reaching down into the trousers of a stranger on a bus and masturbating him to climax

18 \ while you're down there ...

Several themes crop up again and again in women's fantasies:

- Rape
- Anonymity
- Being watched
- Feeling humiliated
- Being stretched
- Sadomasochism
- The forbidden
- Prostitution
- Other women

Mucky little hussies, aren't we? Go forth and fantasize, lady.

> **DID YOU KNOW?**
> Forty per cent of women have had lesbian fantasies. And just over one in twenty females have actually had 'girl-girl' sex.

GET TO KNOW YOURSELF

May I introduce you to ... you: the female of the species. Exploring your sexuality isn't just about having fun with fantasies or bringing yourself off whenever you've a spare moment (though this is a lot of it, obviously). You've got to get to know your own body intimately. Every nook and cranny, every erogenous zone, every hot spot that gets you going. Every spot you know of, that is. The great thing is that you'll never find them all. This is a lifelong learning process that'll very possibly encompass several partners and certainly very many masturbation sessions.

Let's do what we're constantly trying to stop our men from doing and begin by focusing on 'down there'. Later in the book, we'll be exploring all sorts of different places that love a little bit of lustful attention. But to begin with, let's focus on what makes you a lady. Not your table manners and your finishing-school finesse: your genitals. Just think how much men love their penises. Learn to love your bits. They are what make you different from men, with all the sexiness that difference provides. They give you pleasure, joy – potentially even new life through childbirth. Never pick on your vagina, I won't allow it. We're not supposed to be perfectly symmetrical and nipped and tucked like porn stars. If a man ever tells you otherwise, he obviously has more experience of two-dimensional women than three-dimensional ones.

But it probably wasn't a man who maybe turned you off yourself. Is it your own, self-formed opinion? Admittedly, 'vagina' is a pretty ugly word – a difficult-to-spit-out combination of letters, too scientific-sounding to love. When a group of nine- to sixteen-year-old girls were asked to come up with a better word or phrase that encompassed all that this amazing thing does, they came up with 'power bundle', which is none too shoddy.

DID YOU KNOW?

Far from being obscene, the word 'cunt' is Indo-European, derived from the goddess Kali's title 'Kunda' or 'Cunti'. It has the same root as the words 'kin' and 'country'. It's a pretty good word, too. Very hot and powerful. Perhaps we should be using it more in order to reclaim it and take away its negative connotations, its force as a taboo.

Woman: A Tour – The Capital City

I remember a boy's description of his first glimpse of a woman's genitals from a rude book I read and reread during my adolescence. He said it was '... complicated. Lacking the plain lines of my own organ ...' Go on. Get a mirror out. Have a look. It's true, isn't it? It is complicated. It must be daunting for a boy at first. Girls, ask your man to tell you all his feelings on first seeing one ... but I digress. You're supposed to be concentrating.

Take a good look at yourself. Ever masturbated in front of a mirror? It's amazing, seeing your vagina contract again and again as your orgasm pulses through you. If you're not quite ready to face your sexuality in such a full-on way just yet, simply take a look at yourself when nothing sexual is going on, perhaps after you've had a relaxing bath. I bet you find yourself thinking sexy thoughts, though. The vagina is, after all, incredibly sexual in itself. Why else do men's magazines print pictures of it without its owner's face anywhere in view? The very fact of it is a beautiful sight. Take a good, long look. Maybe touch yourself – not necessarily in an arousing way, just explore yourself and your body. This is what you're seeing:

The Pubic Mound

Also known as the '*mons pubis*', this is the layer of fatty tissue over your pubic bone, which protects you from the grinding action of sex – although particularly rigorous grinding can still hurt, as every horny teenager knows. You and your man should stroke it and love it like a pet.

The Outer Lips

Known by technical types as '*labia majora*', these contain erectile tissue and swell when you are aroused. This means that they may well be more sensitive than you perhaps realize. As with everything down there, go gently. Stroke them too, and tease them with your fingers. Get your partner to lick them up and down.

The Inner Lips

The '*labia minora*', unlike the outer lips, are hairless and may be darker in colour – and darker still the more aroused you get. They protect the clitoris and are also full of erectile tissue. They usually have rather uneven lines and come in all sorts of colours, shapes and sizes. They may poke out from between the outer lips or be tucked up and away behind them. Just because they're little, don't ignore them. Delicate lips, tongues and fingers there? Yes, please.

The Urethral Opening

The hole where the pee comes out. Under-explored as an erogenous zone, but stimulation of it is allegedly very hot for some girls. This has led to enthusiastic label-givers christening it 'the U spot'.

The Vaginal Opening

You'll no doubt recognize this as the bit men usually make a beeline for, their cocks drawn to it like a gang of under-age kids to an unscrupulous off-licence. This bit likes tongues and fingers inside it. The first 2 or 3 inches are full of nerve endings which like attention, but only once you're ready for it or you'll get sore. You know unequivocally when you're ready, of course. Being the classy creature you are, you ease any passage inside you by getting wet. That's the big giveaway. On the whole, this is the way your vagina likes to do things, so don't let blokes attempt to stab away at you before then. The pubococcygeus (PC) muscles (see page 100 for further info) are found in a ring just inside the vagina.

The Vagina

In its resting state, the vagina itself heads for 3–5 inches towards the small of the back and is flat. When you have sex, it lengthens and opens out to accommodate your man – although different positions have different effects on it. Doggy style, for instance, has the effect of shortening it relative to, say, the missionary position. This gives your partner the sensation of thrusting deeper into you. The vagina gets wet when it is excited because blood flow to it increases and this provokes a 'sweating reaction' in the vaginal walls.

The Cervix

This is as high up into the vagina as a penis can go and it feels like a relatively hard nub. It is the entrance to the womb and secretes a mucus which protects the womb from outside infection. When a man is inside you, thrusting into you, if he jabs this it is eye-wateringly bad news. Ask blokes (especially big boys) to go easy when they're new to your internal anatomy. Just as men's penises are different shapes and sizes, so too are women's vaginas. The cervix may be off to one side slightly or further back in one woman than the next. Some women love (careful)

here's looking at you / 23

attention to the cervix, but many don't. Gently explore your own responses.

The Clitoris

The clitoris is much larger than you might think: most of it is hidden inside you. The visible part is a pea-sized fleshy knob of erectile tissue. This is located above the vaginal and urethral openings, at the top of the *labia minora*, and is covered by the clitoral hood. The sole function of the clitoris is to give you sexual pleasure – stimulation of it is the most common way for women to come. See also pages 27-8.

The Perineum

The perineum is the area between the genitals and the anus, and it's often neglected on both men and women. Due to the dense network of blood vessels below the layer of skin – which fill up when you're aroused – it's sensitive to careful stimulation. For some women (and some men), the feeling of a vibrator on it sends them over the edge.

The Anus

This is a powerful muscle and it has the second most nerve endings of any part of the body, so it's sensitive. Seems a shame not to make the most of that, doesn't it? If you're up for anal sex (think back to those fantasies again – does the idea of it get you going? Do you fancy giving it a go in real life?), you and your man must have the patience to get it right. Lots of loving attention at first, soft fingers and tongues. And only go for it if you're totally happy with what's going on. If you're uptight and not relaxed in any part of your brain or body, it's going to hurt; if you're calm, however, it can be quite the sexual high. See also page 139.

> ### HOW DO YOU DRESS YOURS?
>
> Inspired by a friend who said that if her vagina got dressed it would wear a red beret, Eve Ensler, the brains behind *The Vagina Monologues*, asked other women what their vaginas would wear. Here are a handful of her favourites:
>
> - A pink boa
> - A male tuxedo
> - Armani only
> - Something machine washable
> - High heels
>
> What would yours wear?

MASTURBATION TIPS

Eighty per cent of women masturbate; 94 per cent of men do (and twice as often). Try varying your routine with yourself. Much as you might whinge about the habits you and your partner have fallen into, I expect you've got routines all of your own when it comes to making yourself come. And if you don't masturbate, please, please do. You'll be bowled over. It will open up a whole new vista of sexual possibility and pleasure to you.

Just because masturbation is between you and your body alone, it doesn't mean you can't or shouldn't be inventive. Allow me to use a food analogy. If you're hosting a dinner party, you'll probably go to town on the menu, rustling up delicious dishes with a tasty mix of flavours and using only the very best ingredients. If you're dining solo, perhaps you just throw together a bit of pasta and shop sauce, or opt for a plastic-tasting ready meal. My advice? Take more care. Value yourself more. Just because it's only you eating, don't serve yourself second best. Just because you're not making love with a partner, don't skimp on the sexual hedonism. Masturbate as though you're making love to the most sexy, most important person in the world. Guess what? You are. Here are some tips:

- Tease yourself – go up, down, around, in, out, shake it all about if you have to. Orgasms are always more intense if they're delayed.

- Use a dildo or a vibrator – but gradually, gradually, getting yourself wetter and wetter, until the whole thing is inside you when you come.

- Watch yourself in a mirror. See if you can hold your own gaze or if you have to close your eyes eventually. Notice your face becoming flushed.

- Talk dirty to yourself – try out all those words you daren't yet with him. You'll feel silly at first, but – oops – see the effect it's having.

- Use a (gentle) clip of some kind to pinch your nipples, perhaps a little hairclip. But go carefully, obviously.

- Try it with an ice cube inside you.

- Bring yourself off on your elbows and knees – rubbing your breasts against the bed or on a couple of pillows.

- Rub yourself against something – perhaps straddle a pile of pillows with a soft toy on top and a towel over that. Ride it, girl.

> **Case Study: Sandra**
>
> *'I was seventeen before I masturbated properly. By that time, I'd already had four sexual partners and I thought I'd had an orgasm ... boy, was I wrong. But I didn't know what I was missing. I'd never brought myself off, so even when lovers turned me on and got me close to the edge, I didn't know how to push myself over it. One afternoon, after I'd finished my A Level exams and was home alone, I put on a sexy video a friend had lent me. Pretty soon, my pussy was throbbing and I was getting wet. Knowing no one else was in the house kind of liberated me, and I began touching my vagina while sitting on the sofa. I wasn't entirely sure what I was doing, I just followed my instincts and did what felt good. When the sensations became all-consuming, I didn't stop, I just kept on going, and going, and going ... till I was gone. A-mazing. I've never looked back since.'*

Okay, time out for your heartbeat to return to normal.

See how most of these tips can be applied to sex with your partner too? Realize, then, how important it is to take time to play with yourself. If you know the kind of thing that gets you going, you'll be able to show him. If you start experimenting by yourself, you'll be confident about it when you begin a new sexual adventure with your lover.

Remember: you should never put something inside your vagina that you wouldn't put in your mouth.

DID YOU KNOW?

Sex using vibrators is most common in Australia and the USA. Fifty-two per cent of Indians said they wouldn't buy a vibrator.

THE CLITORIS – A 'Q+A' INTERVIEW

Tell us a joke.

How do you give a lemon an orgasm?

Don't know.

Tickle its citrus.

Hmm, okay. Perhaps you're best off sticking to your sole purpose of giving women pleasure.

Fine. All the emphasis seems to be on the G spot these days. Freud even described an orgasm produced by me as 'inferior', yet no one is uncertain whether I exist like the G spot, and the vast majority of women need me to be able to come, whether or not they can get off in other ways too. The G spot may even just be stimulation of me by another name and from another angle.

Yes, aren't you much bigger than was first thought?

Yup. Ten years ago they thought the clitoral head – the bit you see if you draw back the skin above it, which in turn draws back the clitoral hood – was the extent of me. All that was really known was that this swelled and became more prominent when a woman was aroused. Actually, I'm more than ten times larger than that, which is why the entire area can become sensitive to the touch during sex.

In fact, I consist of eighteen parts in all. Ian Kerner, author of *She Comes First*, summarizes my far-reaching influence well: 'Stop thinking of the clitoris as a little bump and start thinking of it as a complex network, a pleasuredome, the Xanadu at the heart of female sexuality.'

You're sensitive, right?

Very, very, very. My head is the equivalent of the head of a penis, but it contains twice as many nerve endings – 8,000, give or take – within a far more confined space. So it needs to be handled with extreme care and love. Think butterfly on a fragile flower rather than hammer banging away at a nail.

What else do we need to know?

It's worth bearing in mind that just because I'm small, it doesn't mean I'm not susceptible to and grateful for a range of sensations. Lick me, suck me, rub me, stroke me: it's all beautiful. Keep it coming.

THE G SPOT – A 'Q+A' INTERVIEW

How old are you?

Depends who you ask. I was first mentioned in the West in 1944 by gynaecologist Ernst Gräfenberg. Things went quiet for a few decades and then I was named in his honour by sex researchers Alice Kahn Ladas, Beverly Whipple and John D. Perry in the 1970s. Still, practitioners of tantric sex have known about me all along – they have been calling me a 'sacred spot' for more than a thousand years.

Are you sure you exist?

Well, people are always arguing about my precise nature. I'm still a controversial topic. Not every woman has one of me and Gräfenberg's claim that pressure to me causes female ejaculation is even more contentious. It is in this spirit that you should search for me. Women are complex creatures and your sexual triggers are many and varied. If you start looking for me and decide that I'm not there, and that Gräfenberg, Ladas, Whipple and Perry are all off their heads, I bet you find some other area that heightens your sexual pleasure. As Chia and Abrams put it in *The Multi-Orgasmic Woman*: 'Each woman may have her own pleasurable spots that are just not yet famous.'

So where are you and how do I find you?

I'm between 1 and 2 inches inside the vagina on the front wall, behind a zone which is about the size of a watch face. I myself may start off small – the size of a pea – and then swell to a larger size when aroused. Can you feel an area that's rough like a walnut, rather than smooth and silky like much of the vaginal wall? I'm right behind that. It's much easier to find me if you're already pretty gaga with sexual excitement. Then stroke me, please. The movement to keep in mind to stimulate me is to make a beckoning or 'come hither' gesture, which gently 'grazes' me with your index finger. Mmm.

Please try to focus. What do you do?

Sorry. Sometimes I produce very intense orgasms indeed. I'm highly sensitive and can send some women into new and wonderful worlds of sexual ecstasy, but initially you might just feel the urge to pee when you track me down. Gräfenberg claimed that I cause ejaculation in a woman which is equivalent to that of a man, but these days no one can agree on whether this is a special fluid or just brief, arousal-induced incontinence – I'm right next to the bladder, you see. Either way, research suggests that about 10 per cent of women expel 9–900ml of fluid from the urethra during arousal and orgasm. The very latest thinking is that it is indeed urine, but that the chemical composition of it is altered due to sexual arousal. Aren't I clever?

Nice talking to you. Any other advice?

Yes, actually. Sometimes I feel that people get so hung up on finding me that they forget to enjoy the ride. But if you're not enjoying yourself, you're not going to get the most out of finding me anyway. We are getting too conscientious, which is ridiculous for sex. And sex itself is already too destination-centred with its emphasis on orgasm. I think we should all enjoy the journey more. Then any destination we reach will be a wonderful bonus.

GETTING IT ON

Sex statistics give all sorts of impressions: one survey revealed, for example, that 83 per cent of men enjoy sex 'a great deal', but fewer women do, at 59 per cent. Clearly, this pretty substantial discrepancy is something that needs to be rectified as soon as possible. Speaking of which, as far as sex goes, there are a number of changes that we women might consider making to our mindsets, to make our sex lives that much more successful:

- **Empty your mind.** Get rid of any assumptions you may have about your partner and what sex is for. Don't assume he won't fancy you if you've got your period, are pregnant or are stuffing yourself with banana fritters. And remember: sex is your friend; it can be employed in almost any circumstances. In love? Out of love? Premenstrual? Tired? Headache? I prescribe a dose of sex for all of the above. Knowing the First Secret of Successful Sex, which I will deal with later, will also help you enormously.

- **Have confidence in your body.** When women are troubled, we talk. And we talk more about body shape and body image than anything else. But we are our own worst enemies. It was the tabloid picture-editor's wife who noticed Diana, Princess of Wales's cellulite when she was photographed leaving the gym. Stop being small-minded about others and you'll soon apply the same rules to yourself – and cease to be thrown into a depression because you don't wake up airbrushed every morning. And if you feel good about your body, you'll want sex. Come on, you know this.

32 \ while you're down there ...

- **Show him the dirty you.** It's there, as you almost certainly know from the thoughts you have when you masturbate. What's all that trust for, if not for this? Show him he's met his mucky little match. If talking dirty doesn't come naturally to you, do it on your own when you touch yourself. Think you'll feel stupid? Try it – it works. And remember: he's not out to find fault with you. He won't peer over the top of his half-moon specs and criticize your talking-dirty style – he'll get a raging hard-on and give you a damned good seeing to.

> ### FAKING IT
>
> If you're not yet ready to reel off a list of instructions in bed, start by not lying. That means no more faking orgasms. Nearly half of women recently surveyed in the States said they had faked orgasms. How patronizing. How is your sex life meant to evolve if you are being dishonest about something so fundamental? And no more holding on to simmering resentment, either. Introduce honesty into everyday life and it will carry over into sex. Say if you're angry. And compliment him if he's getting it right.

What Kind of Sex Would You Like?

So what, in your wildest dreams, will it be tonight?

- **Slow, lazy, sensual sex.** Taking-your-time sex; sex with a scented candle lit, perhaps after a tasty meal, maybe featuring asparagus, oysters and chocolate. Lots-of-kissing-to-get-you-going sex. Perhaps, if you even decide to go for penetration, in the spoons or hands-free position (see page 96).

- **Hard, fast, urgent sex.** Sex to undo the week's stresses; sex that drives all other thoughts from your mind. Perhaps you'll manage it standing up. Perhaps he'll bend you over and do you from behind without even undressing you properly. Giving-it-to-each-other-and-collapsing-in-a-panting-heap-afterwards sex …

- **Intimate, quiet, sexy sex.** Introspective, no-words-allowed, concentrating-on-feelings sex. He might want to explore you thoroughly. You've got all the time in the world, but if it's that sexy, sensual and intense, I bet at least the first orgasm comes sooner for you than you expected. Take a quick rest and you'll soon be ready for the next course – luckily for us, most sex is like that for a woman. We can keep going all night with regular rests and a willing partner.

- **Dirty, up-for-it sex.** One of you drives the other crazy by telling them a nasty, sexy story … until he can't keep his hands off you any longer. Perhaps the first round will be a bit of a wham-bam-thank-you-ma'am affair and the second something more dangerously deliberate. Perhaps you'll keep doing it like bunnies, all night long.

- **Curious, educational, we've-never-tried-this-before sex.** Get your toy box out. Don't have one? Establish one (see page 146). This is sex involving: 'Ooh, what do these beads do?' 'Let me squirt a bit of this on to you and then put them up there.' Or, 'If I switch this on and put it there, it looks so good. What does it feel like?' Pushing-your-own-boundaries sex. Trying-something-you-read-about-in-a-magazine sex.

34 \ while you're down there ...

Let's go and get you some of these. And if you're not sure where and how to begin, all will be revealed between the covers of this book.

Read on for some explosive experiences ...

WHAT HAVE YOU LEARNED?

You're home alone with a few hours to spare. What do you do?

- **a)** Use the time to work out to your favourite aerobics video, over and over again. You've just got to get rid of that huge bottom of yours.
- **b)** Recline on the bed with just your libido, your fingers and your filthy imagination for company. You shouldn't need three guesses to know what happens next.
- **c)** Reorganize the kitchen cabinets, wash every single item in your partner's wardrobe and give the house a full spring clean. You want everything to be perfect for your man.
- **d)** Study a saucy magazine that tells you exactly how to give a great blow job. You might not have had an orgasm for three years, but it's paramount that you satisfy your man in bed.

chapter two
the art of communication

You're feeling sexy, secure and safe in the knowledge of your newly awakened sexuality. But it takes two to tango. It's time to look at your relationship with your man.

> **DID YOU KNOW?**
> In a room of fifty couples, it takes the average woman less than fifty minutes to assess the relationships in the room. In the same amount of time, a man has slightly improved his aim throwing peanuts into the ashtray.

Whether we like it or not, and regardless of the fact that we should obviously be treated equally, here are the headlines: men and women are different. This leads to the best and the worst things about sex: difference is exciting and exotic; but the different don't always understand each other.

You'll have heard this a million times before, but ... sex is a mode of communication. It all starts and ends with communication. There is barely a relationship on the planet that could not benefit from better communication. But many of us, perhaps taking our cue from our parents, never learn to communicate properly at all.

Add to this our conviction that if someone loves us, they'll 'just know' what our needs are and it isn't surprising that we find ourselves in a fix. The if-it's-right-they'll-know-instinctively impression is instilled in us from the very first. When we were young, our parents – in fact with a limited number of options and a lot of guessing – seemed to know what we wanted without us having to tell them. So:

Love = Automatically knowing what I want

Yet adult relationships cannot work like this. Your partner isn't going to know that you love that thing he does with his tongue unless you tell him. You can't expect him to guess that you hate it when he rolls over without making you come just by huffing and puffing and giving him the silent treatment. A good sex life has its foundations in a strong relationship; a strong relationship is built upon effective communication. Learning to communicate more successfully with your partner – on all levels – naturally leads to a reinvigorated sex life. That's what this chapter is all about. Forget about the actual sex ... just for the moment. If you and your man are failing to address issues in your partnership, the chances are that the relationship is rocky in areas beyond the bedroom. Your shaky sex life may simply be a symptom of more deeply rooted difficulties.

LOVE OR LUST?

Firstly, though, have you identified what kind of relationship you're in? We often confuse lust with love, especially initially, and we do so over and over again, even in the face of clear evidence that a relationship can be loving without great sex and vice versa. Perhaps it's because, as far as brain patterns go, that initial, passionate feeling of falling in love is similar to having a mental illness, such as obsessive compulsive disorder.

By all means try to base your relationship solely on that heady, dizzy, 'in love' feeling – good luck to you. But the feeling of being 'in love' is largely based on novelty and old-fashioned lust, backed up by a tradition of romantic love.

Scientists have determined that lust's neurotransmitter is dopamine – in the right quantities this acts on the brain to create energy, exhilaration and focus. In other words, the feeling that we experience early on in a relationship is just a kind of chemical high. It's never going to last, so there's no point in yearning for it or over-sentimentalizing it. Usually, a major factor in a sex drought in relatively new couples is the inevitable end of this initial infatuation: it endures for only 3-12 months, or at the max for two years, depending on whom you ask. It certainly doesn't last a lifetime, anyway. I think this is partly because it takes considerable effort for men to seduce women. Infuriatingly, they cease to expend that energy as soon as they can. The skills we associate with seduction – talking and listening, say – come much more easily to women. It's just the way our brains work.

One solution to the problem is to make a man believe that he hasn't seduced you yet. This leads to the fairly tedious situation we've all seen – and perhaps participated in – where people break up to make up the whole time: the on-off relationship. But that's not relating to each other and it doesn't lay a foundation for anything – happiness, say, or a future, or being able to have a life outside of your relationship.

Another, more successful, approach is to take an interest in our differences, to understand better where we're missing each other. Clue: it's probably happening on a daily basis and you're putting it down to other things – his wilful tendency to undermine you and be selfish, say, or (to his mind) your inability to be rational and to treat him as anything other than a failure.

In fact, most of us are being kind and considerate in our own language – it's just that we need to learn another. It's that old chestnut communication again, but these days, finding out more about the brain as we are, we stand a real chance of being able to achieve it; and then everything between a man and a woman, including sex, should improve. We can just continue to roll our eyes heavenward, of course, but it won't lead to more fun in bed.

HARDWIRING – MEN AND WOMEN

A simple fact that has long been ignored is that men and women communicate differently. This is not a New Age, touchy-feely theory: it is a fact about the way our respective brains work. For a start, men are simply not as adept at conversing as women. MRI scans show that when a man has a conversation, the whole of the left hemisphere of his brain is employed in finding a centre for speech. In women, the centre for speech is found in very specific areas on both sides of the brain, which leaves the rest of the brain free to do other things. In other words, if men

> ### Case Study: Lucie
>
> *'Whenever I'm annoyed with my boyfriend, I immediately call my best friend for advice. It helps me to talk through the issues with her and get some feedback. But Simon gets angry when I phone her first – he thinks I should go straight to him with any problem. I know he's right, really, but sometimes it feels like he doesn't take in a word I say. He assures me differently, though, and his actions usually back that up. Yet it's hard not to seek out my best mate's sympathy, when he always seems so preoccupied when I try to talk to him.'*

don't appear to be listening and responding, it may be partly because it's harder for them to do so.

Women have also evolved a huge range of listening expressions. To show that we're listening to someone, we use around six expressions per ten seconds. We also change our body language and intonation. Given that men haven't necessarily got these tools at their disposal, it's easy to see why women end up whinging about their men to girlfriends who listen, rather than talking directly to partners who appear not to.

DID YOU KNOW?
Men are chiefly concerned with getting results, achieving goals, status, power and beating the competition; women care about communication, cooperation, harmony, love, sharing and relationships. Sometimes it's surprising we can relate to each other at all.

Did you know?
The bit of the brain that handles emotion is in two parts: the 'temporal limbic' part deals with sex and aggression; the 'gyrus cinguli' is linked to thinking and imagining. Guess which sex is geared towards which?

What is a Conversation?

A straightforward question, you may think, but you and your partner will probably have very different viewpoints, which suddenly renders discussions potential minefields of misunderstanding. Ever raged at a partner for trying to 'solve' something you're saying, rather than listening and empathizing? That's because, for a man, talking is primarily a functional thing rather than a bonding thing. He likes to think something through in his head and then express it. When you air your thoughts to him, he thinks you're asking him to work through your problems in the way that he does his, when in fact you're simply sharing information. For women, speaking is thinking aloud and being inclusive, an apparently rather formless process of letting the other person know where we're at and how we're feeling. It concerns itself more with the journey than the destination – women are like that about most things, come to think of it, especially sex. For a woman, the ideal upshot of a conversation is to feel understanding and understood; for a man it's to find a solution.

So, if you're trying to convey something and are just getting back weird, solution-sodden replies, it's not because he thinks you're hopeless and incapable of thinking for yourself, it's because he's trying to help you reach the conclusion he believes you're after. His urge is to find solutions to what you're saying; if that doesn't go down well, that's when he says that things don't matter. He doesn't realize he's undermining you in saying this, he simply doesn't know that in speaking to him you're trying to reach him and get his support.

These different approaches often lead to failures in communication. When he seems casual, you think he doesn't care. His emotionless mask is off-putting and to all appearances cruel. But his unwillingness to show his feelings is just a hangover from the days when he was worried about the proximity of sabre-toothed tigers to his cave, but felt single-handedly responsible for making the family feel that everything would be all right. Seeming casual and emotionless is probably the way he has always gone about things, in every single relationship he's ever had. Don't take it personally.

Remember, too, that men can find it difficult to discuss information they're not comfortable with. Relationships, sex and feelings – matters that will very likely come up in your conversations as a couple – are the very topics that may cause him to feel overwhelmed or, as the counsellors have it, 'emotionally flooded'. Don't force it. It'll just make him run and hide. If a man shuts off, you should let him do it: he'll be fine. You might find it easier to broach the subject in bed with the lights off: not, you understand, using sex as a one-size-fits-all bandage, but using the cover of darkness to liberate him. He'll be much more likely to open up if you can't see his face. If there is a problem between the two of you, you may find that he skirts around the subject and ends up addressing something entirely separate.

Are We Really Saying What We Seem to Be Saying?

The fear of communicating about essential matters afflicts both men and women. Sometimes, we tackle too shallow a demand with our speech. 'I wish you'd wash up' can actually translate as 'I wish I felt more supported' – it's just that we shy away from dealing with the real problem. Both of you should work on avoiding expressing a trivial problem in place of a deeper one. Be honest about what you're thinking and feeling. Don't tell him

---

THEY FUCK YOU UP, YOUR MUM AND DAD

Your blueprint for interaction is your parents' relationship. Of course, some people react against their parents and emerge completely different from them, but the vast majority of us will act out in later life what we witnessed earlier. Got a sullen partner who won't talk to you? I bet his parents were either always shouting at each other or the house was quiet, but filled with a hostile atmosphere. Either way, his response was to withdraw – and it still is.

As far as developing into an evolved human being goes, the best atmosphere to have been brought up in is one that was not completely harmonious – because you learn nothing about conflict resolution in that instance. When the shit hits the fan, what do you do if you've not been taught how to deal with it? No, far better to have witnessed a relationship that, when conflict arose, reckoned on sitting down and resolving the dispute, rather than sweeping it all under the carpet.

you wish he'd take the bins out more often when the genuine issue is that you feel you're collapsing under the weight of the whole relationship and you need some encouragement and help. Unsurprisingly, he thinks everything's fine, but you just wish he'd take the bins out more often.

DID YOU KNOW?
Under pressure, men act without thinking and women talk without thinking. This leads to conflict – it's inevitable. 'What did you do that for? Talk to me.' 'Can't you just shut up for once in your life?' and so on.

TALKING TO YOUR MAN: A HOW-TO GUIDE

DID YOU KNOW?
Relationships often fail because of men's reluctance to talk. In the UK, getting couples to complete communication exercises forms the vast bulk of the work of master relationship counsellors Relate.

- If you want to communicate information to a man, keep it simple. Many women can keep up with several topics of conversation at once; although men exist who can do this too, on the whole it's best to stick to one subject at a time – an approach everyone can follow.

- Don't tackle topics obliquely like you would with a woman – he'll never pick up on what you're talking about. Be direct. And use short, no-nonsense sentences like he does, or he'll lose the thread. While we're about it, are you one of those people who – especially after a bottle of wine – uses very long, rambling sentences, followed by: 'Am I making any sense?' Answer: you're not. Not to anyone. Male or female. A good friend will tell you so. If you just want to be listened to, never ask that.

- Be literal – and don't use language that's too emotive or he'll fail to compute. If you tell him he never listens or that you never have sex any more, he'll just think, 'Yes, I do,' or 'Yes, we do.'

- Don't use 'can' and 'could' requests – he'll feel both that he's being forced to do something and that you're implying he might not be capable. Unless you've landed yourself an uncooperative bastard, 'will' and 'would' should work a treat.

> **DID YOU KNOW?**
> If you want instant access to the inner life of a man, listen to the song he's singing/humming/whistling to himself. There it is: his subconscious right there for everyone to hear, whether your critical faculties want to or not.

- Allan and Barbara Pease, authors of *Why Men Don't Listen and Women Can't Read Maps*, say that if you want to make maximum impact on a man, you should tell him what you want to talk about and when. They also recommend that you give your man an agenda, but that would sound a little scary to my partner – especially if there were two or more things on that agenda. Simply keep things clear and concise, and if you want him to listen rather than offer solutions, tell him that in advance.

OLD HABITS

Partners can take terrible liberties with each other when they've been together for a while. Assumptions abound. And where there is assumption, there is rarely good news or anything very exciting or creative going on.

There are wonderful – and potentially very rude – things about having been together for a long time; being known well can be a joy. But there is no joy when each of you believes you know *all* there is to know about the other.

In day-to-day life, we tend to stop inviting or expecting intimacy. We start to function. Questions emphasize doing rather than feeling: 'How was your day?' rather than 'How are you doing?'

We often think we know what our partner's saying when we don't. This is extremely irritating for them, as it gives the impression that we can't be bothered to listen to them, hence that we don't care. In fact, we do care very much. Partners for the most part want to make each other happy. Both of you just have to work on helping each other to understand how.

- When a man says he'll think about something, he probably will. He's not just procrastinating or, worse, disinterested. He'd simply rather have a conversation with himself first, come up with a response and then let you know what it is.

- It's hard to swallow, this one, to say the least, but a good way to communicate with your man is not to interrupt him. It sticks in the throat because, in conversation,

76 per cent of interruptions are made by men. There must come a point when self-respect steps in for a woman, though. If he's being an overbearing bore who's making it up as he goes along, I say interrupt away.

- It's hardly ever worth employing 'the silent treatment'. It's a waste of our short time on the planet and men don't notice for five minutes. Hilariously, Allan and Barbara Pease warn that he may even come to think of the silence as 'a kind of bonus'.

DID YOU KNOW?

Taoists say that it takes seven years to know your partner's body, seven years to know his mind and seven years to know his spirit.

TAKING STOCK – A RELATIONSHIP EXERCISE

Is there a larger problem that needs addressing? Are you placing the emphasis on sex – when actually there's something deeper going on?

Without wishing to be a spoilsport, it has to be said that most of us are mindless optimists when it comes to new relationships. Initially, we think that – at last – in our new partner we've found the perfect person to answer all our needs. Being misunderstood and dissatisfied has magically become a thing of the past.

Time passes. Disillusionment can enter. Surprise, surprise, your unreasonable expectations are not met after all. You might start doing miniature, secret, cost/benefit analyses in your head. Is this worth it?

the art of communication / 47

In a spirit of enquiry and interest – and on the basis that knowledge is usually a very good thing – together or alone, complete the following exercise. Think about what annoys you about your partner, and your partner about you, and write any issues down.

Common niggles may include:

- How close one of you is to another person – or to friends and family in general.
- The amount of personal space you or he is getting.
- The amount of time you spend together.
- Not showing affection.
- Feeling the other doesn't take responsibility in the relationship.
- Not feeling romantic or sexual any more.
- Not respecting each other.
- Not having enough fun.
- Feeling undermined by the other.
- Feeling subject to the other's moods.

Are any of these familiar? It's not terminal ... yet. Remember: the best environment is not one where problems are absent, but where, when problems inevitably crop up, they are dealt with properly, rather than badly or not at all. So let's look at solving these issues.

How do you react to any of these or other obstacles that you come up against in your partnership? Be very honest with yourself here, rather than defensive. We can all construct a version of our behaviour that frees us from blame completely – but this fails to move things forward.

Here are some common responses. Do any of them accurately describe your or your partner's approach?

48 \ while you're down there ...

- Being open to suggestion.
- Trying to be honest and clear.
- Keeping calm, and keeping a sense of perspective when you discuss things.
- Retaining a sense of humour.
- Encouraging the other to talk by asking questions.
- Listening and being constructive.
- Trying to talk about feelings.

Or do you:

- Sulk
- Raise your voice
- Leave the room during an argument
- Clam up
- Shout
- Rake over old coals
- Blame the other
- Talk over the other or talk too much
- Fail to look at the other
- Change the subject when you sense a sticky topic arising?

THE FIVE-MINUTE CONFESSIONAL

The MTV-generation alternative to the exercise on page 46 is the five-minute confessional. With the help of an alarm clock, each listen to the other for five minutes and then swap over. Just make sure you then deal with whatever problems crop up: a task that might take a little longer than five minutes ...

Have a look at your list of issues. Are these problems big and insurmountable – or are they small and things that you can work through together? Of course, there are ways and ways of working things through …

HOW TO HAVE A ROW WITHOUT WRECKING YOUR RELATIONSHIP

- Tip number one: criticize cleverly. A friend once shared with me something he was taught on a management training course. He had his tongue firmly in his cheek as he described it, but for all its silly jargon, I respect and understand what it's getting at. His course told him that the secret to successful criticism was the 'feedback sandwich' – meaning that if you want to get the best out of someone, you tell them something positive, then the bad news, then something else positive. For example, 'I love it when you kiss my neck; hate it when you make no attempt to find my clitoris; love it when you make me a cup of tea in the morning.' Or something like that.

- Secondly, remember that being able to appreciate someone else's feelings and opinions is at the core of most successful relationships. In order to be able to do this, we have to exercise a degree of self-control. Calm cajoling is a more effective tool of persuasion than tantrums and brute force. When did aggression last work as an approach to motivation? Instead, practise non-threatening communication. Ditch the battle responses. Don't tell him he ruined your evening; tell him you didn't enjoy the evening. Use even, calm tones when you express yourself.

A NOTE ABOUT KNOWING WHEN TO CALL IT A DAY – SEX AND SULKING

It struck me, during the course of writing this book, that there are times when partners are trying to get it on, but are coming from such different sides of the planet that day – mentally and spiritually speaking – that they should give it up. Not walk-out-the-door-and-never-come-back give it up, you understand, but recognize-that-sex-can-wait-until-tomorrow-or-we'll-end-up-in-an-argument-and-hurt-each-other's-feelings give it up. Put the kettle on, or criticize his selfishness and undermine his sexual confidence for ever? Hmm. Your choice.

- Listening is what keeps couples together. If your partner is heatedly criticizing you, your automatic response will very often be to produce the defensive rebuttal: this treats the criticism as though it's a personal attack, rather than an attempt to change things for the better. The enlightened listener will let the criticizer finish – difficult as this may be – and try to identify the cause of the outburst. This is empathy in action. Once the angry half of the couple has finished, you should edit out the hostile, personal aspects of their diatribe and calmly ask for clarification if you are unclear about the real substance of it.

- Good listening is active. Employ responsive facial expressions to let your partner know that you're absorbing what he's saying. Your body language should signal approachability: face him with your arms open, not folded in front of you, and don't slouch. This in turn will help you to listen, in the same way that simply smiling can often make you feel happy.

- Relationship guidance counsellors encourage 'mirroring', which is the reverse of what goes on in problematic heated discussions between couples, where partners take opposing sides and begin a slanging match. 'Mirroring' is expressing back to your partner what he's trying to convey to you, perhaps adding an assessment of your own about how you think it makes him feel.

A CHEAT'S GUIDE TO COMMUNICATION

- Beware misinterpretation. If you're not absolutely sure what your partner is saying, check with him.
- If you want to take, you have to be prepared to give.
- Whenever you are negotiating, start small.
- Honesty, honesty, honesty. Without this, there is no partnership. If you're happy, tell him. If you're angry, express it openly. Never bottle things up or fail to communicate a new emotion to your partner: it'll only fester inside you and eventually ruin the relationship.
- It takes time for a person to drop their guard. If you and your partner are trying to be more frank in general and about sex, be patient. You may need to practise.

SHOULD I BE WITH THIS PERSON?

If your rows are occurring on a regular basis, however, and communication has suffered a major breakdown, you must ask yourself this key question. It's one thing to try to enliven a sex life if there's a relationship worth saving, but sometimes the sex isn't working because there's a much more significant problem: the two of you are fundamentally mismatched. Put the following questions to yourself, to determine whether it's worth attempting CPR on your sex life, or whether now's the time to cut your losses and leave.

1 Is this person my friend?

Have you chosen to be with someone you wouldn't pick as a friend? A surprising number of people do this. Just stopping for a moment to think about it might save a lot of heartache and a lot of wasted time.

People often form an ideal type in their heads and then seek out an approximation of that. Men might choose very outwardly glamorous – but emotionally unstable – girls, who their female friends (not so glossy, easier-going) don't get on with. Women might choose macho men who are horrible to them, when all their male mates are talkers and 'new men'.

Then what do you know? Instead of talking to the people who need the information, i.e. their partners, about the (inevitable) problems they're having with them, both the men and the women end up discussing these with their friends. Of course they do: they get on with them! I've had several male friends like this, to the extent that I have to suppress a giggle each time they ring up and suggest a drink. I know they've had a row with the girlfriend they shouldn't be with and their solution is ... to spend time with a 'safe' girl they feel they can talk to. Bonkers.

2 Does this person make my life better?

Another simple question often ignored by people in their haste to couple up. In my experience, being single has a lot going for it. You're not answerable to anyone; you're truly free; anything's possible. And being with the wrong person is a huge waste of everyone's time. Hear this: the person you're with should keep you feeling free. Nothing else is good enough. Pay attention to me. Hold that thought close. Check they do.

Like most simple things, this is an easy point to lose sight of, but ask yourself: is this fun? Because this is all there is. You're doing it now. There's no magical time in the future when everyone will change and everything will be fine. If things are at a status quo and you're miserable now, it ain't gonna alter all of a sudden. Sit yourself down. Face these things. Don't put it off. Talk to your partner about them.

3 Do I trust this person?

Yes? Wonderful, because this is the true foundation of a healthy relationship – and, by extension, of good sex, incidentally. What if the answer's 'no'? Well, first establish if the lack of trust is your doing or his. Are you the jealous type? Is emotional baggage from your past getting in the way? Are you a pain in the arse about trust? Perhaps he's constantly trying to reassure you and you won't hear it? Or are you right? Has he been unfaithful? If you search your soul and you know he's untrustworthy, get out of there. If

54 \ while you're down there ...

you search your soul and find you've got trust issues – and you can ask a friend if you're still not sure: tell them to be honest, and be prepared for them to tell you if you have a problem – then seek help from a counsellor (see page 155).

Keep It Simple, Stoopid

If even the above questions seem too much like hard work, but you're feeling ultra honest and want some frank answers on the status of your relationship, just consider your partnership and ask yourself one simple question:

Am I happy?

If you've answered 'yes' to all of the above, yet are still plagued with doubts, take heed of Martha's wise words:

> **Case Study: Martha**
>
> *'I have a message for those who habitually wonder if the right person is just around the corner and the person they're with might not be the right one after all. I have a great relationship with my husband, but will confess to having wondered at regular intervals if I shouldn't be with the last man I had a good chat with. After several years of this, I've finally learned to sit myself down and tell myself this: "Martha. Do you seriously think that after six months or a year this person is going to be any easier to live with than your husband?" Simple, but wise words for those with a wandering eye.'*

WHAT HAVE YOU LEARNED?

Having said he would, your partner has failed to take the bottles to the bottle bank for two weeks running and it's really got your goat this time. What do you do?

a) Send him an email with the subject heading 'Re: You're a filthy pig', which says: 'Absolutely typical. You never try to help me out in the house and I've got a book which says I have to tell you when I'm angry ...'
b) Take the bottles to the bottle bank yourself, biting back your anger and fantasizing furiously about the man you met in the pub the other day. After all, your new book says you should fantasize more and your revenge can be to store up these images for use in bed later.
c) Resolve to raise it later, calmly, along the lines of, 'Would you take the bottles to the bottle bank?'
d) Leave the bottles be and ring your friend to bitch about him and his unreasonable behaviour for half an hour or so, so that by the time he's home you're over it and he never knows anything about your wrath.

chapter three
the sex factor

Okay, so the lines of communication between you and your partner are open and fully operational. Now is the time to reintroduce the sex factor. Sex brings with it at least as many quirks and additional considerations as there are people to contain them, and some of these quirks may result in inhibition or communication problems between lovers. So they're worth addressing, in order to diffuse any difficulties.

We all have our own, deeply felt hang-ups about sex, usually as a result of past experiences. It's worth exploring these before we even broach the subject with our partners. For example, where did you first pick up information about sex? In the playground, where the intelligence was probably riddled with inaccuracy; in the classroom, where only the technicalities were discussed; from the movies, which consistently fail to portray sex authentically? What was your family's attitude towards touching? Were they natural and loving about it or did they hold back? Did you ask them how babies were made? Did they palm you off – or make you cringe?

FACING YOUR FEARS

The best way to deal with any sexual quirks is to face potential problems head-on. The idiosyncracies that we all possess are often solely in our heads. Think about it: why do we rarely ask our partners directly what they want? There's a simple answer: we fear what would emerge if we did. After all, with sex the response won't be merely, 'You're not supportive enough' or 'I wish you were more of a conversationalist,' we fear it will be 'I don't fancy you any more,' 'I fancy X more than you' or 'You just don't satisfy me.' Ouch.

Ouch and, of course, rubbish. Unless your relationship is all but over or you picked a malicious bastard,

---

YOUR WORST FEARS

What are your worst fears about expressing your sexuality to your partner? Write them down. If you confess to getting off on thinking about doing it in a veterinary nurse's uniform with six strangers, or any of the fantasies on pages 16-17, what will he do?

a) Will he dump you?
b) Will he jump you?
c) Will he say 'yuck' – and then find himself thinking about it obsessively at work and flushing a little when he does so, unable to believe that he's landed such a filthy minx?

Who knows? Except that I assure you it won't be 'a'. It's got to be worth a go, hasn't it? I dare you.

your partner will not be feeling these things, he will be thinking about what the two of you could be up to and worrying about whether he's getting it right. So don't be afraid to communicate with your man where sex is concerned.

The Ex Files

It's hard to talk about sexual history with a partner, but this might be something you're hung up on. Perhaps you're constantly comparing yourself to his ex, or are worried that you're too experienced/not experienced enough. Either way, it's stopping you from committing fully to your current sexual relationship.

If you *really* think it would be useful, work up the nerve to ask him about his past or to bring up yours. But beware opening the can of worms that comprise 'the ex files': neither of you may like what you find.

On the other hand, much as we all fear being told that we're not the best, most uninhibited lover he's ever had, in reality I don't think our sex lives are that dissimilar between partners. So you shouldn't worry too much about the Ghosts of Bedrooms Past. As a friend once reassured me when I was bitterly imagining my revitalized ex with his new, Swedish girlfriend: 'You know, he's probably pretty much the same as he was before.' 'Good point,' I thought ... and if that's enough for her, then good luck to them.

As a general rule, you should avoid comparing yourself to others. Whether you think you're better or worse, at the end of the day it's just a distraction from the exciting task at hand. I used to know a girl who had always felt threatened by what she perceived to be the incredible sexual exploits of her best friend. The friend was very noisy in bed – everyone had heard her – and she had a special kind of smugness on the subject of sex: a smugness that said, 'Now, that's something I'm rather good at.'

One day, Inadequate Friend got talking to Sexual Athlete's first boyfriend. 'All that noise she makes, it's not real, you know,' he volunteered matter-of-factly and apropos of nothing. 'It's pure theatre and it's for everybody else's benefit.'

DID YOU KNOW?

Women ogle men just as much as men ogle women, but we have better peripheral vision so we get away with it.

MEN VERSUS WOMEN: A ROUGH GUIDE

- Thirty-seven per cent of men think about sex every thirty minutes; 11 per cent of women think about it as often.
- Women average nought to orgasm in thirteen-and-a-half minutes. Men average nought to orgasm in two-and-a-half minutes (once penetrative sex has started). (But it could be worse: an African baboon mates for only ten to twenty seconds, giving just four to eight thrusts per mating.)
- A woman's sex drive increases as she gets older, reaching its peak in her mid- to late-thirties. A man's sex drive peaks at age nineteen or twenty and declines gradually from then on. Seasonally, both men and women peak in autumn – in time for babies in spring/summer.
- On average, a woman's orgasm consists of six to ten contractions and a man's of four to six.

> **DID YOU KNOW?**
> In our twenties, we have sex about 148 times a year; in our thirties, 110 times a year; in our forties, 78 times a year.

KNOWING ME, KNOWING YOU

Keep up the excellent communication we established in the last chapter. Don't go all coy on me now that sex has entered into the equation. If you're going to ask for what you want in bed, you and your partner need to be honest with each other in every regard.

Most likely, you're a bit shy about conveying your deepest, darkest sexual secrets. Contrary to what one might think, there is a sense in which the longer you've been with someone, the harder it gets to talk to them about intimate stuff. It matters, after all. What will he think? Of course, it doesn't matter really. He'll love the fact that you're opening up to him and sharing your filthiest thoughts. He might even surprise you with his response.

As you know deep down, the best way of overcoming a fear is to face up to it. No need to dive in at the deep end just yet, however. Instead, here's a quick quiz to ease you into opening up to one another.

Do this exercise with your lover, completing the following sentences about your partner's, and then your own, sexuality:

- Your favourite place to be touched is …
- The quickest way to make you come is …
- You like it best when I …
- Your favourite position is …

WHY SEX IS GOOD FOR YOU

Not that you need any encouragement to leap into bed with your man, I'm sure, but here's the scientific bit that proves we should all be at it like rabbits:

- Endorphins (feel-good hormones) are released into the brain during sex, which activates the body's opiate receptors. As well as giving you a fantastic natural high, they are nature's pain relievers and good for helping with, among other things, whiplash, headaches and arthritis. This gives a scientific foundation to Richard Wilbur's bold yet accurate claim in *The Observer* that 'Most women know that sex is good for headaches.'
- Having sex three times a week burns off around 35,000 kilojoules. Apparently, this is the equivalent of running 130km in a year. So if we up our – for most people – two sessions a week by just one, we can consider ourselves not only more sexed-up, but athletes into the bargain.
- Sex increases testosterone levels, which is good for bones, muscles and good cholesterol.
- DHEA (dehydroepiandrosterone) is released just before climax. It aids cognition, helps the immune system to operate efficiently, inhibits tumour growth and strengthens bones.
- A woman releases oxytocin (love's neurotransmitter – see page 63) during sex and this too is associated with better bones, as well as an improved cardiovascular system.
- Overall, these hormones also protect the heart.
- Put together, all these benefits result in a longer life. So get to it!

62 \ while you're down there ...

- I think the best way to turn you on is ...
- You think the best sex we ever had was ...

- My favourite place to be touched is ...
- The quickest way to make me come is ...
- I like it best when you ...
- My favourite position is ...
- The best way to turn me on is ...
- I think the best sex we ever had was ...

Now compare notes. Did you find out anything new? Are you up for implementing these things? Have I lost you because you're already trying? Excellent, excellent.

DID YOU KNOW?

In *New Scientist* magazine, Professor Stuart Brody of the University of Paisley found that penetrative sex was particularly effective in reducing the stress levels of people about to speak in public.

A ROUGH GUIDE TO MEN AND SEX

- Because men can be a bit crap at multitasking, they sometimes can't talk during sex. Because we women are nest defenders, we can't always switch off during sex.

- Like a rooster, a man can only make love to the same chick five times a day (lucky you if his cock can perform better than this).

- He jokes about sex with his mates not because he doesn't take sex seriously, but because if they spoke frankly about it, each guy would have to start getting his statistics out and then someone would be the loser.

DID YOU KNOW?

Love's neurotransmitter is oxytocin, which in the right quantities is a bonding drug – sometimes known as the 'hug drug'. Prairie voles mate for life and have high levels of oxytocin. If their oxytocin receptors are blocked, they stray. When one of us becomes more attached than the other, as like as not our oxytocin levels are mismatched.

- When men channel-flick or read newspapers and fail to pay attention to a word you say, they are not just being lazy, incommunicative arses. According to the discipline socio-biology, they are harking back to a time when they would sit in front of a flickering fire and relax after a strenuous day's hunting. (These days, he might want to consider that by doing this he's also failing to adhere to the First Secret of Successful Sex, of which more later.)

- Men's testosterone comes in five to seven waves a day. It is at its highest peak at sunrise – when he gets his morning glory, and you're sometimes woken by a 'broom handle' in the small of your back – just before he sets off for a day's 'hunting'. It is 30 per cent lower in the evenings when he is 'fire-gazing'.

- The average strokes-to-climax figure of a masturbating straight man is 62, compared with a gay man's 58 strokes. When asked what measures they took to clean up, 394 men used their hand, 73 used an old sock, 141 used a hanky, 12 did it into the sink and 43 used a plant pot. The survey also recorded that 806 felt intense joy after climaxing; inadequacy and gloom were experienced by 201 participants.

- He probably doesn't remember that stunner in the green dress who was flaunting herself under his nose at the party. He might have caught the odd curve here and there, but then he'll have forgotten all about her. His attention span isn't that protracted: there's beer to be drunk, ball games to discuss ... His eyes take it all in, but it doesn't register in any significant part of his brain.

- His biological make-up is such that he wants to provide for you. If you appreciate this, he feels like he's a success – like he's fulfilling the job description.

- Men worry about being seen as failures; they're much more likely to ask for directions when you're not there. And they need to feel capable of solving their own problems. If you try to help, he'll think you're implying he's incompetent, which is why he clams up. If you can make him think something was his idea, he'll be much more receptive to change.

- Take heart. Far from obsessing about other women, most men measure their sexual prowess according to your sexual pleasure.

- Your man finds you physically more attractive if he's in love with you. He rates you lower in attractiveness if he doesn't care for you.

DID YOU KNOW?

Seventy-seven per cent of attached under-thirties are very satisfied with their sex lives; compare this to 53 per cent of their single counterparts.

PUTTING THE LOVE BACK INTO LOVEMAKING

Sometimes, we can forget to do this very simple thing. Gorged as we are on a diet of sex secrets and often unfathomable how-to guides, the 'love' part of lovemaking can fall by the wayside. The pressure to be 'good in bed' (whatever that means – it's so subjective), coupled with all the other social demands that women face daily (the pressure to be a career girl, mother, domestic goddess, fashionista and friend, for example), means that we occasionally approach sex with a focus and ambition better suited to the workplace. Relax. This is between you and your man. This is about your feelings for and attraction to each other. Nothing else. There isn't going to be a six-month appraisal and a salary review. He's not grading you out of ten. Though it's fun and important to try new things in bed – that fabulous vibrator you've just bought or a new technique you read about in *Cosmo* – it's essential to remember why you're there in the first place. Sex isn't just about orgasms and heady heights: it's about real emotion and expressing that in an incredible, beautiful, sensual way.

You and your partner may not appreciate (or may have forgotten) how important romance can be. An interesting, little-known fact is that women who read romantic literature have twice as much sex as other women. Over time, sex becomes an extension of how we feel about our partner in other ways. We may start to take our partners for granted in bed. Yet none of us knows each other inside and out sexually – there is always more to learn, both about your own desires and your partner's. The key is to view each other as sex objects again; to recall what it was you fancied about each other in the first place – or what you've found attractive about them over time.

Romance Tips

- The traditional options are no less effective for having been used in the past: cook him a meal, serve it candlelit, play soft music and end up making love. Or go out to dinner to your favourite restaurant.

- Dance with your partner whenever you get the opportunity. In the kitchen as you're tidying up; whenever a significant song comes on the radio; at weddings or in nightclubs; in a shopping centre or elevator to the piped Muzak.

- Recreate your courtship rituals from the early days of your relationship. In doing so, you can revisit all those early exciting feelings too. It really works.

- Dirty weekends. Those couples who continue to have them tend to thrive while others fall by the wayside.

- Think yourself sexy: by thinking about positive aspects of your partner and the sexiest experiences you have shared with him, you can arouse both yourself and him.

- Every day, bear in mind the all-important First Secret of Successful Sex (see page 154).

> **DID YOU KNOW?**
> Jazz fans have 34 per cent more sex than pop fans. If classical music's your thing, you're probably having the least sex of all.

Sensual Massage

Most of us get out of the habit of massaging each other after the initial infatuation phase of the relationship has passed. It's one habit we should get back into. The desire to be touched is a human one – and who should be doing it to us if not our partner?

1 Begin by setting the scene: burn aromatherapy oil and candles scented with rose otto, jasmine or vanilla. Dim the lights. Both of you remove your clothes and any jewellery. Perhaps put on some relaxing music (preferably not pan pipes). Lie your partner on the most sensual fabric you have ... that you can afford to get oil on. If you really want to heighten his enjoyment, you could blindfold him with a silk scarf (the woollen ones don't work so well). The sensation of your touch will be magnified as he loses the power of sight.

2 Pour the oil you're using for the massage straight on to your partner's skin, rather than on to your hands first.

3 Begin at the base of the back with your hands splayed and facing your partner's head. Use gentle strokes up either side of his spine and up over his shoulders and along the tops of his arms ... and then move down in one long, slow, sweeping motion. You'll eventually finish with this motion too.

4 Introduce some kneading, interspersing the use of your thumbs and fingers on his muscles and flesh with long, slow, sensual strokes up his spine. Use the flat surface created between your first and

second knuckles when you make a fist. Don't knead too hard – it's supposed to be sensual rather than chiropractic.

5 Go with the flow and stay focused – and he'll be in heaven whatever you do. Make sure you keep in contact with him throughout. Lose yourself in what you're doing and concentrate only on the feel of his skin beneath your hands. If it's love action you're after, mix in some teasing: a fleeting bit of attention to his butt cheeks here; a bit of reaching round his torso or a few butterfly moves on the back of his neck there. Or nibble him – gently. Perhaps give your man's massage an extra kick by oiling up your breasts and massaging him with those. Hear him moan – in a good way – when he figures out what's going on.

6 Make sure you swap over after you've taken him to seventh heaven and back. This is something you *definitely* want reciprocated.

DID YOU KNOW?

Once women feel special in a relationship, they have more orgasms – two or three times as many in monogamous relationships; four or five times as many when married. There is also an increase in your orgasm rate once your partner tells you that he loves you.

MAKE LIKE A CRAZY WEASEL

Proteus was a Greek river god who had the advantage of being able to evade capture by changing his form at will. One minute he would be an animal, next a tree, next a cloud. Evolutionary biologists have applied this story to adaptation in animals and called it 'protean behaviour'. If you're a rabbit, behaving unpredictably – by running in zigzags – stops you being eaten. If you're a weasel, doing a crazy dance baffles your vole, enabling you to pounce on and eat it. Author Geoffrey Miller, in his book *The Mating Mind*, applies this same theory to successful relationships: 'Whenever one animal [is] able to predict something about another animal's behaviour or appearance, the second animal might benefit from making its behaviour or appearance unpredictable.'

In other words, don't get stuck in a relationship rut. Shake up your routine every now and again – in every way. Get your hair cut, buy some new clothes, initiate sex, suggest a new pastime that you and your partner can pursue together. How about some paint-balling sessions? Or taking up ballroom dancing? Every now and then, change something simple about yourself or your routine – and you'll have him falling in love with you all over again. If you evolve, your relationship will too.

Case Study: Donna

'I'd been going out with James for three years when we hit a bit of a rocky patch. We weren't rowing all the time or anything like that – it was worse, we didn't seem to have anything to say to each other, angry words or otherwise. The whole relationship just seemed a bit boring, in all honesty – there was no spark from either side. Really down in the dumps, I decided to sort myself out and booked a spa weekend for just me. It gave me time to sort my head out. I had some beauty treatments, facials, massages and so on, and came back with a spring in my step and a lighter heart (and a whole new wardrobe: sometimes the only way to celebrate is to go shopping). James was delighted to see me – he said me being away had made him realize what he felt for me. We went out for dinner that night and talked for hours. Not just about our relationship, but about everything. It was brilliant to have my best friend back. After that, we knew we were on the right track. And the next time I arranged a weekend break, we went together.'

Mutual Masturbation

If you've made yourself come on your own, tell him about it. The notion of him masturbating's sexy, isn't it? Imagine what it does for him. When you're masturbating together, tell him exactly what you're doing and how fast or slow. Get him to do the same. If his account is making you touch yourself faster, tell him so.

Oh, and when you come, look at each other, if you don't already. It's amazing.

Seven Great Sex Myths

I'd advise against attempting any of the following sexual shenanigans. Whether you're wanting to spice up your sex life or simply try new things with your partner, these are not the starting points of the savvy seductress. Some of them are recommended by so-called sexperts and raved about by certain magazines – you'll undoubtedly have come across them before, if not in your own sex life, then certainly in the media or on the World Wide Web. Just because something is hyped, however, that doesn't make it hot. My experience is that these sex myths are *so* not worth the effort. By all means try them if you want to – but I may not be able to resist the urge to say, 'I told you so,' when the whole thing dies a disappointing death.

The 69

This position presents each of you with the other's genitals from about as unhelpful an angle as could be. Ideally, he needs to be able to get at you from the bottom up rather than the top down; ditto you to him. Also, it's difficult – if not impossible – for the two of you to concentrate simultaneously on what's being done to you and what you're doing. And if one of you is on top, you can't use your hands because you need them to support yourself. Avoid!

Doing It in Front of the Fire

Two sets of two words: carpet burns; scorched flesh.

FIVE BAD REASONS FOR HAVING SEX

1 Revenge. You want to hit back after your partner has done you wrong (as you see it): maybe he was unfaithful, or flirted with someone else, or simply failed to notice your new look. 'I know, I'll have third-rate sex with someone else,' you think – and almost instantly regret it.
2 Pity. 'He was so up for it and I've been so tired and grouchy recently, I thought I'd go along with it.'
3 Reward. People who give or take away in order to punish or reward their partners are known in the psychotherapy trade as 'withholders'. Don't have sex to get rewarded, either. Some people share a 'we-both-know-if-he-gets-his-way-he'll-give-me-his-credit-card-to-play-with' attitude. Grow up. And get a job of your own.
4 Duty. 'We haven't done it for ages; he's starting to take it personally; let's get this over and done with.'
5 Power. Unless it's some kind of pre-agreed S&M (sadomasochistic) deal, don't have sex with someone to demonstrate the emotional or physical hold you have over them. If you're a halfway decent person, you'll feel like shit afterwards.

Doing It in Water

Not only tricky logistically, but dangerous. The water washes away natural lubrication and may cause you internal damage. Plus condoms don't work as well, being prone to slipping off.

Girl-on-Girl Action

A famous rapper once said that any woman was only a couple of Sea Breezes away from a threesome. He should have added 'with a famous rapper'. While it's true that we women can be truly ravenous sexual creatures, put simply, wanting to do it with a woman must involve wanting ladies' bits. If you go for girl-on-girl, but don't have a passion for pussy, you're simply being a man-pleaser.

Sitting on His Face

Don't do this. Please – there's no point. He can't manoeuvre properly or use his hands on you; or see what he's doing, in fact. You're going to get very sore thighs from kneeling down on either side of his face – which is what you're actually doing – taking the strain so that you don't crush his skull to smithereens.

Doing It Standing Up

What are the chances of you both being the same height, or him being strong enough to hold you on to him?

Threesomes

He'll want it with two girls; you'll want it with two men; the one who doesn't get their way will end up feeling left out ... or the third person will, which rather defeats the purpose of having a threesome.

While we're about smashing myths to pieces ...

Pregnant Sex

Not a lot of people know this.

Until they come out, everything about babies is good for the libido: making them, having sex while they're gestating.

First there's making the baby: fantastic, no-contraception-necessary, intense, kicking-up-your-heels-and-going-for-it sex. Both of you experience this primal sex-for-its-original-purpose feeling. And the rules are that you keep doing it all the time until you're pregnant ... oh, go on then.

Then there's the pregnant sex. No one tells you how horny you get while pregnant – it's all that extra blood flow to the nether regions. And if you're, say, writing a sex book at the time, which entails reading about sex, poring over erotic fiction and road-testing sex toys, the effect is even more extreme. Ridiculous, almost.

It's true that towards the end you might have some trouble performing some of the more athletic bedroom manoeuvres and, in truth, shifting your huge bulk around at all, but these problems can be surmounted if the will's there. And the will's there.

Top four positions for pregnant shagging:

1 Doggy style
2 Hands-free (see page 96)
3 Spoons
4 You on top

What's that? You're wearing him out, you say? Urge him to read some erotic fiction; watch porn with him; use sex toys on him. Tell him your dirtiest fantasies. This is your last chance before you're robbed of the rest of your life by a tiny tyrant who would rather you never had sex at all.

DID YOU KNOW?

Research shows that the average time for making love is 10.34 p.m.

FIVE GOOD REASONS FOR HAVING SEX

1 Because you're horny.
2 Headache.
3 Period pains.
4 To help an insomniac get to sleep.
5 To celebrate that it's Wednesday.

WHAT HAVE YOU LEARNED?

You've just got together with a new partner and are keen to make a good impression in bed. What do you do?

a) Set aside an evening dedicated to each other's sensual pleasure, cooking a meal with aphrodisiac ingredients, treating each other to aromatherapy massages and so on.
b) Challenge him to try it standing up and against a wall. To show your commitment, you'll have chosen the wall in advance.
c) Ask him to describe his past lovers, to demonstrate that you're an open-minded person who's

76 \ while you're down there ...

> completely cool with his previous experiences ... until you ruin that impression by bursting into tears when he gets to the naughty anecdote about the Brazilian exchange student.
>
> **d)** Lie back and think of England, without communicating anything about your own desires.

chapter four
let's get it on

Are you feeling just the tiniest bit horny yet? I bet you are. All this talk about sex without actually getting down to the nitty-gritty of nookie, the hard-and-fast facts about fucking, the ins and outs of intercourse. A tease, *moi*? But here it comes at last: a no-holds-barred how-to guide to getting you the best sex you've ever had. Life will never be the same again, I promise.

You already know I'm not a proponent of blame. It doesn't achieve anything and it certainly won't improve your sex life. Accusation leads to nothing but love lost. Nonetheless, your man and his approach to sex are major players in the sex-quality stakes. I'm guessing he's not just an animal or you wouldn't be with him, because that would be illegal; he probably laughs along sagely as women crack jokes about men who can't find the clitoris. But he still:

- Places too much emphasis on the act.
- Can't shut up about anal sex.
- Has ceased to see you as a red-hot sex object.
- Doesn't know the First Secret of Successful Sex.

He needs to focus on you again. You must get him to want to be an expert on you, fostering a near-scientific interest in your responses and responding to them with the flair and attention of an artist. He must become a brilliant artist/scientist hybrid – an aficionado, possibly in a white coat if it does it for you (see 'Fantasies for Sharing' section, page 127).

WOMAN: A TOUR – THE WHOLE COUNTRY

Your man should begin by taking his time over your whole body, as though it's a precious thing he's seeing for the very first time. Can you recall when he saw it for the very first time – and how exciting that was? Try to recapture that same, breathless feeling. Focus on the fact that we can never know everything about our lovers – the tantalizing potential of the unknown does still exist between the two of you, however long you've been together. You've barely scratched the surface and yet think you've uncovered everything, when you're only at the tip of the enormous iceberg that is each other's sexuality.

Let's go back to your body. He might notice new things about it as he meticulously explores you: a freckle here, a little scar there, the way you gasp if he runs his fingernails lightly down there. Why not suggest he strokes your hair, or touches your back and traces the lines of your legs? Get him to move his hands gently over your belly. He should stay in slow control, teasingly avoiding the obvious bits – I bet you're a melting, enchanted thing already, aren't you?

Erogenous Zones

Now let's take things a step sexier. Having *too* conscientious a lover or getting too hung up on erogenous zones ruins things for everyone, but that's not to say you shouldn't both try to find them – in fact, I'd recommend it. Erogenous zones vary – and move – from girl to girl, and are also affected by your mood, who you're with, where in your menstrual cycle you are and what's gone before. There's lots of fun to be had in searching for those special places that drive you (and him) wild. On a good night, the whole body feels like an erogenous zone. With an attentive lover, the following are all contenders for the title – and, of course, triggering a few of them has a knock-on effect, bringing the more blatant zones to life.

Feet

Never underestimate the power of a good foot massage – and don't forget each individual toe and the tops of the feet. Start off gently and increase the pressure. Both sexes will enjoy some foot fondling: a very macho ex of mine once got a huge hard-on from another friend of his as a result of a good 'un. I don't think he ever recovered. The masseur should ask what feels good, because some people like firmer pressure than others and some are incredibly ticklish. Don't be absent-minded. The foot massage, as well as being downright arousing in its own right, is also an excellent transition to sex. One minute you might be watching TV, the next you've got your eyes closed and are en route to ecstasy.

Backs of Knees and Inner Thighs

Two obvious places to which to proceed immediately after the foot massage. Your bloke should take his time here, however tempted he is to try and rush on into you. This is about seducing you. Tell him to work his way up slowly, teasing as he goes ... you'll be completely ready for him by the time he reaches the top. If he makes you wait, I bet he'll already have blown 99 per cent of the male opposition out of the water. Am I right? You're never going to forget him. You're his for the taking whenever he chooses.

Underside of Your Arms

As a pick-up artist once observed, with women the underside of everything is the most sensitive – including the breasts and buttocks. Before your man gets on to those main attractions, however, he should concentrate on your arms, using the tips of his fingers and brushing the skin with his lips – but not too lightly, or it'll just be irritating and make you itch.

Case Study: Sarah

'There's a point on my neck that is the most sensitive part of my entire body. I've never known anything so responsive; I didn't know my body could be that responsive. It's just at the top of my spine, a hard knob at the base of my neck that I can feel if I roll my head forward. If my partner kisses me there, even if I'm just standing at the sink doing the washing-up, it sends blood rushing straight to my cunt. It is such a turn-on. My boyfriend's started using a vibe on me there after I've had an orgasm. It sets me off again immediately, and I'm just there writhing around on the bed, riding the waves of ecstasy, all because he's touched this tiny little bit of me. I've never known anything like it.'

Neck

This is so hot, but somehow on a man's mission to get inside us, he often forgets it – fool. It's such an oversight, because some well-targeted neck action is a direct route to being 'ready' for most girls. He should use his lips and the tips of his fingers at the same time and – gently, gently – flicks of his tongue and the slightest pressure with his teeth and … mmm.

Ears

Ask your partner to journey here via your neck. Beginning below and behind your ears, he might then start to nuzzle your ear lobes, pulling at them gently with his lips and his teeth. Beware of licking, which can be off-putting – of course it's loud, he's just by your ear! Persuade him to whisper sweet nothings or talk dirty to you – and swoon.

Hands

When the time feels right, plunge one of your fingers into his mouth and get him to lick it at the same time. A degree of disorientation works wonders with sex and this will remind both of you what you'll do to him when he gets inside you. The palms of the hands contain tens of thousands of nerve endings too, so don't ignore them. If he buries his mouth in your palm and licks away, he'll give you a delicious foretaste of what it'll feel like when he goes down on you.

Abdomen

During foreplay, I think little teasing brushes with the backs of the fingertips work wonders here. Men and women both love the lightest of flicking sweeps with a fingernail up or down, just below and parallel with the bottom rib.

Next, command your man to begin mixing the journey around these spots with visits to some of the more tried-and-tested, familiar areas, which are flushed and ripe and ready for him now, unless I'm very much mistaken ...

TANTRIC KISSING TIPS

I would recommend all of these tips, but only once things are already pretty hot and heavy:

- Suck each other's tongues and lips (one lip at a time).
- Explore each other's faces with your tongues – including the eyelids and under the chin, which is an especially sexy zone.
- Put fingers in mouths. While you kiss, slip your finger(s) into the other person's mouth. This is incredibly erotic.
- Put mouths on fingers. Specifically, kiss, lick and suck the sensitive skin between the fingers and the thumb itself. Men, in particular, love the thumb thing: it's highly sensitive and reminds them of being given a blow job.

Lips and Mouth

Ridiculously sensitive, these, on both of you, so don't just kiss them, nibble them lightly, catching one then the other in your lips; lick them a little – just teasingly. Touch them. Toy with them with any part of your body you can think of. Don't go straight into a clumsy, high-school French kiss, but when your tongue does begin exploring inside, and as the intensity increases, gently touch the roof of your lover's mouth with your tongue.

Face

Despite Hollywood movies to the contrary, this is, regrettably, a rather under-explored zone. Perhaps it takes a special degree of courage that other parts don't demand, to look into someone's eyes and touch their face. At the very least, while you're kissing, try exploring the texture of the skin on your lover's cheek with your fingertips – and ask him to do the same. Both men and women adore it, as it feels so personal and direct.

Breasts

As you'll know, a whole variety of approaches to these can get you going, but you might want to mention to your man that he should avoid tweaking and sucking them at the very beginning. As he starts to fondle you, go gently: suggest he brushes the undersides of your breasts and the sides, where they hang over your ribs if you're lying on your back. Ask him to lick and then blow on them. Tease, tease, tease. He should save the serious grabbing and nipping until you're really aroused and even then go carefully – neither of you wants a reality check when you're in the throes of passion.

Bottom

I think it's great to have your hips or your bum cheeks grabbed by your lover when he's inside you. Before then, though, don't ignore this highly sensitive part of the body – on either of you. Run your hands down your lover's back and finish by cupping his buttocks firmly, squeezing them with your whole hand. In return, ask him to knead, squeeze one of your buttocks in each hand, spread the cheeks – and then continue on his erotic quest.

By now, he'll be trying to ignore your gasps of ecstasy, which make him want to pin you down and give it to you there and then. Both of you: hold on. It'll be worth the wait, I promise. Once you finally reach your climax, long postponed and all the more passionate for it, you'll be able to think of little else all day tomorrow – and for the rest of your life.

DID YOU KNOW?
Of 1,000 female students, 96 per cent favoured cunnilingus over penetration. In another survey, just 3 per cent of men, and 6.5 per cent of women, disliked oral sex.

CRIB NOTES FOR A PHD IN CLITERATURE

Despite what the movies show, all the sex surveys ever undertaken suggest that the number-one way to get a woman off is through oral sex. Whatever form this takes, I imagine you're highly unlikely to complain about your partner making love to you in this way (unless what he's doing is painful). In the interests of creativity, eroticism, self-expression and not paralyzing your man's jaw, however, it's an idea for him to vary his technique a little. It never hurts for him to have a few more tantalizing tricks up his sleeve.

CHOOSING THE RIGHT TOOLS

As Ian Kerner, author of the excellent *She Comes First*, observes: 'Making love with one's penis is like trying to write calligraphy with a thick magic marker.' He's talking specifically about arousing a woman, not intercourse itself, and he's got a point. Your man wouldn't use a wrecking ball to knock a picture hook into place now, would he? (Well, not unless he'd been watching too many demolition shows on TV.) The same applies to the process of making you come. The tools he needs here demand exactitude, sensitivity and responsiveness. He must have mastery over them. Does his manhood measure up?

Very often, the answer is no. And it's nothing to do with size, you understand – or even premature ejaculation. It's the accuracy we're most interested in. So when a man makes love to you, don't exile his erection from proceedings, but encourage him to employ his mouth, tongue and fingers with finesse. You love the visual pleasure of a hard cock rubbing up against you and your clit loves the general sensation, but a wet tongue burrowing into blissful hidden crannies simply cannot be beaten.

Let's assume he's already got you ready with a long, languorous sensual massage and a lot of kissing and licking ... everywhere but on your vagina. Your face, neck and chest are flushed and you're pretty wet for him by now. He must ignore his cock as it screams 'Get inside her! Get inside her!' Its time will come. For now, he's going to use his mouth on you to send you away with the fairies.

And unlike some men, he's going to finish the job. Perhaps you've had lovers in the past who abandoned you partway through, giving the impression that they'd grown impatient at your lack of climax. You might be worried about taking too long to come, but any lover worth his salt will a) not give a damn about the time it takes to transport you to heaven and b) be more concerned about getting you there any which way he can. Trust me, he won't have a stopwatch down there. The time will be the last thing on his mind. Think about it: he's face to face with your fanny. What do you think is going through his head: the passing of time or your slick, wet pussy? Added to which, as we all know, women on average take around six times longer to come than men. He's not expecting it all to be over in minutes and is more than likely grateful that he gets the time to enjoy you and your reactions. He's got all the time in the world when it comes to luxuriating in you. He relishes the process of giving just as much as you relish receiving it. Relax.

Cunnilingus: A How-To Guide for Men

If you can persuade your partner to read this section himself, so much the better, but if you feel a bit shy about being so upfront, then make subtle suggestions next time you're in bed together. Though not *too* subtle, of course – you really don't want to miss out on any of these moves!

1 First, get comfortable.
2 Lie so that the two of you are in a long, straight line.
3 Your partner might want to rest his forearms on a pillow, so that his hands can reach you easily but his

arms won't get too tired. If he can move your legs around and slide his hands underneath your bottom, you're probably in the optimum position.
4 He should be able to put his face to you from where he's lying. This ensures that all the work isn't left to his tongue alone.

Whole books have been written about cunnilingus. I recommend that you seek them out if you and your lover are interested in expanding your routines. To get you started, however, here are a handful of techniques to experiment with, combine, stick to and/or discard, as your moans of satisfaction and his comfort dictate.

'Hello' Kisses

He touches and kisses your pubic mound through your knickers, then attends to your abdomen and thighs. Open your legs a little and allow him to kiss your lips. Only at this stage should he take your knickers off and announce his arrival straight to your pussy – with slow, deliberate kisses down there and perhaps one good, long, slow lick from bottom to top; perineum to clitoris.

Cat Licks

Homework: watch a cat wash itself. Notice its thoroughness and how absorbed it is in its task. Get your man to emulate that, working his way over the whole of your genital area using short, repetitive licks. Leave the clitoral head till last and then – as Ian Kerner puts it, in characteristically beautiful style – 'like a cat that's come across a trouble spot that demands a bit of extra attention, apply more focus and pressure'.

Brushstrokes

Also known as ice-cream licks, these are broad strokes with the tongue, perhaps such as the one he may have used to say 'hello'. They are made with a flat, wet tongue, licking from the perineum right up to the clitoris. They mess you up most if he mixes them with other techniques. There may come a time when he needs to stick to a rhythm, but not at first ...

A Spelling Test

He keeps you open with his thumbs and then spells out your name, or his, or that of his last girlfriend on your clitoris ... you won't give a monkey's what it is, as long as he doesn't stop. Perhaps he'll lick the alphabet on you. If he's really mean – or particularly likes being ignored – he might ask you to tell him what he's writing. You'll be studiously failing to answer his question, your head thrown back and your mouth open, before you know what's happening.

The Clitoral Suck

Once you've become very excited, and only then, he can draw back the clitoral hood, put the whole of the head in his mouth and give it a single – *gentle* at first – suck. He should return to this as part of the mix, perhaps when his tongue is getting tired, increasing the pressure a little with each suck. You're going to come soon, I bet ...

The Clitoral Blow Job

Pretty self-explanatory. As above, but he doesn't move away from you to try other techniques. Instead, he gets a bit of a rhythm going and flicks his tongue around the head of your clitoris – at the same time as sucking it, if he can. Challenge him to show off and combine this trick with using his fingers on and inside you: he'll turn you to jelly.

Flat, Still Tongue

Good for when all his cunnilingus tools have been given a thorough workout and one or both of you could do with a rest, but it's too soon in his plan to stop completely or abandon contact with you. He puts his tongue against the entrance to your vagina and lets you move against it as you will for a while.

Eating with His Fingers

He traces the path of his exploring tongue with a finger. For you, the contrast of the soft and hard should prove pleasingly disorientating. Either with or without using his mouth on your clitoris too, he might move the tip of his finger round and round the entrance to your vagina; or put two fingers or two thumbs on either side of your clit and rub round and round on the shaft as he licks the head; or do the same thing with one hand while holding you open with the other; or, with your clitoris in his mouth, move his head swiftly from side to side while thrusting into you with his thumb; or do that cool thing you love which he invented himself; or, or …

He Nose Best

With his tongue inside you, he moves his nose round and round on your clitoris. He might think what he's doing is absurd, but you won't have a clue what it is – you'll just know how it feels. And you'll want him to memorize it for ever and not stop now.

Obviously, there comes a time when your lover will have to get into a rhythm and let you come, rather than perpetually teasing you and changing the pace for the rest of his life. But you should both remember, too, that delayed gratification leads to the most powerful orgasms. Get the balance right between you – and get ready for a lifetime of sex elevated to another level, with some seriously explosive responses.

> **Case Study: Dave**
>
> *'It's not always men who need finesse lessons. Once, right at the beginning of a relationship, I went down on my new girlfriend for the first time. I set about immersing myself in her body and its responses. After a while, the girl propped herself up on her elbows and said in a loud, harsh, unimpressed voice: "It's all right. I'm up for it enough now. You can fuck me if you like." Instead, I made my excuses and left.'*

Does your lover also know about …

- **The perineal pinch.** It doesn't sound very sensual, but a finger stimulating the tissue just inside the perineum can work wonders. If, with short or blunt nails, he combines this with a thumb in a gentle pinching action, it can feel so good.

- **The gum press.** Sounds and probably looks less romantic still, but who cares when it works like a dream? He raises his upper lip and presses his gum to the very sensitive area just above the head of your clitoris – he'll be stimulating your clitoral shaft. Seeing as he's so advanced now, this gives him lots of scope to use his tongue elsewhere.

- **Pausing for effect.** I'm sure he'll have worked this out for himself by now, but for a really mind-blowing effect, he should get into a rhythm with any one of the techniques explained above and then break off for a moment ... before returning to it. In that brief moment, your whole world will fall apart and bits of your body will go into spasms of shock, but it will be worth it for the exquisite pleasure of his return.

- **Pressing your legs together just before you come.** Despite what you may think, having your legs spread is not the position most conducive to orgasm for most girls. It's a physiological thing – it's easier for our pelvic muscles to begin to spasm if our legs are straight. Get your man to manoeuvre himself so that when D-Day arrives, your vagina contracts around his thumb and his tongue is on the head of your clitoris. Heaven.

Go forth and experiment!

DID YOU KNOW?

A man shouldn't stop when a woman starts coming. His orgasm reaches a point and then he's satisfied; a woman may well keep coming for a while and if he stops his stimulation of her, he ruins the whole thing. A man should be guided by his lover. And guess what? After a rest, she'll be ready to come again. And again. And again ...

PASSIONATE POSITIONS

Coital Alignment Technique

Contrary to the vast majority of porn and Hollywood movies, as far as penetration goes, the ultimate for most women is to achieve stimulation to the clitoris at the same time as a penis is inside her. In the 1990s, American psychotherapist Edward Eichel recognized and tackled this by devising the Coital Alignment Technique.

Like so many good things, the Coital Alignment Technique requires care and practice. At its root lies the missionary position, but it is modified to take into account the satisfaction of the woman. There is no thrusting, and with patience the man can achieve virtually constant stimulation of the clitoris with the base of his penis. Sounds good? Here's how to do it.

1 The man begins by positioning himself on top of you, as though in the missionary position but with his hips slightly higher up your body. Your bodies need to be very close for this to work, and more of his body weight rests on you than with other positions.

2 You wrap your legs around his and rest your ankles or feet on his calves.

3 Next, he puts just the tip of his erect penis back and into you. His shaft, meanwhile, is on the outside, pressing against your pubic bone.

4 From there, the motion you create together is a slow, deliberate, rocking one: up and back, up and back.

5 You need to be moving forwards and up rhythmically with every stroke, to help his pelvis to rock and to

get that penis further inside you and the stimulation to your clitoris.

It'll take time to master, but with persistence you will get it right, and you'll know once you're in the groove: his penis will be further inside you at one end of the motion and pushing the clitoris with its base at the other end. Patience and time are the watchwords here, with this slow, sexy and female-centred position. Practise, practise, practise and you'll be glad you did.

DID YOU KNOW?
In the US, blondes are a bit less likely to have an orgasm than other women, and a bit more likely to have faked it.

Ten More Positions for Clitoral Stimulation (and Their Variations)

1 Missionary

You don't need me to tell you how to do this – nor how either of you can reach down and stimulate your clitoris while you thrust.

You might not know the half-missionary, though:

- You lie on your back with your hips raised slightly (try a pillow underneath them).
- He kneels, twisted a little, so he has one knee on either side of your left leg.
- With his left hand, he lifts your right leg and holds on to it.

- You keep your left foot on the floor.
- He enters you at that angle with his chest pressed against your raised right leg.

It's deep, it looks good for him – and feels a bit different because of the new angle – and you or he can stimulate your clitoris manually.

2 Inverted Missionary

This has lots of other names, including The Swimmer, but the principle is the same for all of them.

- First you jump on top and, with your knees on either side of his thighs, put his penis inside you.
- Then you gently shift so you're lying on top of him and both of your bodies are aligned all the way down. His legs are together and yours are on top of them.
- You move up and down his body, varying the position as you both see fit: you might want your legs apart and his together, or his apart and yours together.

This position allows your clitoris to grind against him with the pace and pressure you choose. It's also good for a tired man if you've been indulging in a marathon session, because if your legs are closed, his penis has some support.

3 Doggy Style

As I'm sure you know, this has possibilities for both of you as far as clitoral stimulation goes – although he'll need good balance to be able to thrust into you using only one hand for support at the same time as leaning forward to get at your clit.

You'll also be getting different sensations to your downward-facing breasts: either of you can reach them for a quick fondle, or you can rub them on the bed or against a pile of pillows, or across the other guy you've brought home ... Positions with him behind are generally pretty good for access to all the bits that count.

4 Standing Up from Behind

You have to be approximately the same height for this one.

- He approaches you from behind, in a wood, perhaps, where you're leaning against the trunk of a tree, maybe holding on to a couple of convenient branches.
- He gropes your breasts and body from behind like a good partner should.
- He lifts up your skirt – you're wearing no knickers, of course.
- You do it urgently, like wild animals, him clasping your breasts in one hand and massaging your clitoris with the other. Lovely.

This is a very sexy position indeed, which is not for every day, but is perfect for the occasional quickie on the way back from the pub.

DID YOU KNOW?

Some couples prefer to have sex while the lady does a headstand. It reportedly gives her a special, light-headed orgasm.

5 The Hands-Free

By contrast, this is a pretty chilled, slow, languid position – also gorgeous, but in a completely different way.

- He lies on his side.
- You lie on your back at right angles to him, with your knees bent over his hips.
- He enters you from this sideways position.

This is great from a dextrous, roaming-hands point of view, because both of you can reach your clitoris and as many breasts and balls as you like. You can't kiss, but with the benefit of a bit of distance you can have a good look at each other's faces.

You can thrust him further into you by reaching between your legs and pulling him towards you, or by propping yourself up on your elbows and thrusting your pelvis towards him. If you're feeling really athletic, you can swivel round into spoons or doggy style.

6 The X

You can't see each other or kiss with this one, so maybe it's best for when you both feel like drifting off into your own little worlds for a spell.

- You get on top of him with your feet on either side of his hips.
- You put him inside you.
- Then you lean back until you reach the bed, being careful not to let him slip out.

There's not much room for manoeuvre or macho thrusting here, so this is one for a pause between more energetic bouts of sex. You might both want to touch yourselves or each other in this position for a bit and contemplate what's just been, as well as planning what's next ...

7 The Starfish

What might be next is this position, much like the one before, but without the manual stimulation and with lots of scope for grinding your clitoris against your partner.

- Both lie on your backs with your heads at different ends of the bed.
- Both spread your legs wide, you with one of your legs under one of his, and the other over, so that he can penetrate you.
- Hold hands to make a rocking motion possible.

Like the Coital Alignment Technique, this allows for constant pressure to the clitoris. Get into the right groove together, take your time and you'll be away.

8 Ultimo

- You lie on your back.
- He kneels between your legs, takes hold of your calves and hooks your knees over his elbows.
- He pulls your hips up off the bed (grrr) and puts himself into you.
- Now he controls the thrusting by moving your legs to a rhythm.

Stimulation to the clitoris will be manual and the lady's doing here, but it is great for constant G spot stimulation.

And you've got to love anything that involves that rocking motion – which you can encourage by rotating your hips.

> **DID YOU KNOW?**
> Seventeen per cent of women regularly achieve multiple orgasm.

9 Swivel

- You get on top and put him inside you, getting a bit distracted from the matter in hand by riding him like the big stallion you see him as ...
- You then swivel to face away from him, being careful to keep him inside you.
- He admires your beautiful back and bum.
- You control the thrusting, despite his efforts to, and might want to shift position so that you have a knee on either side of him.
- If you can balance cleverly or he can prop himself up, or if that second guy you brought back hasn't yet gone home, your clitoris can get a look-in too.

And finally, if all this isn't enough for you and you're feeling ambitious – and he's pretty bendy for a guy ...

10 Sit-Down Sex

- He lies on his back and then swings athletically up on to his shoulders and back into that pedalling exercise position, with his bum in the air.
- Facing away from him, you lower yourself on to his bent-back penis by sitting down on his bottom.

- His heels rest on your back.
- Your hands reach back on to his thighs for balance.

This is not one for the faint-hearted!

> ### SPOONS
>
> Nothing to do with your cutlery collection: the sexual position of 'spoons' is in fact so called because of the close fit of your bodies when you make love in this way. This is a very sensual position, more conducive to slow, smooth, intimate lovemaking than to hard-and-fast fucking. Some couples like to do it this way first thing in the morning, when you're both barely conscious but are feeling horny; or in the middle of the night, when you half wake up to the delicious presence of your partner's naked body.
>
> How to do it:
>
> - You both lie on your sides, with your back pressed against your man's front.
> - He enters you from behind.
>
> The full-body contact of this position is lovely, enabling you to cuddle and caress each other with freely roaming hands. He might want to fondle your breasts; you can reach back to grope his bottom – or simply hold on to your pillow and enjoy it. Sometimes this position forces your legs close together at the top, putting pressure on your clit and heightening your pleasure as you thrust back against him.

DID YOU KNOW?

When you've got your period, you're unlikely to see very much blood if you have sex – and your partner is very unlikely to end up with blood in his mouth if he goes down on you. Women are clearly meant to have sex when we're menstruating because many of us get extra hot for it during that phase of our cycle – and it helps with our period pains. Even if there is blood, we all need to stop being repelled by something so entirely natural. Besides, making love to a menstruating lady is supposed to feel extra lovely for a man.

KEGEL MUSCLES

As every Thai girl who ever did a floor show involving ping-pong balls knows, the key to continued hot sex throughout the life of your relationship (and beyond) is actually well within your reach – and control. There's no need to hand yourself over to a doctor for surgery that makes you look or feel 'tighter', or for your man to opt for an op that claims to enlarge his penis, however – please, please, not either of these.

The secret to an eternity of hot sex for both men and women, but in particular for those women about to have a baby, is to exercise your 'love muscles' with kegel exercises. The 'love muscle' for women is also known as the pubococcygeus (PC) and for men it's the bulbocavernosus (BC). The more toned yours is, the more control you'll have during sex and the better sex will be.

To find these muscles, have a pee and notice which muscles you use to stem the flow. Those are the fellas. They are the same muscles that are weak in incontinent people. In fact, incontinence doctors recommend stopping and starting your pee as one useful exercise to help overcome incontinence. You can do the same, but you're strengthening the muscles for a very different reason.

A PC Workout

Your PC muscles form a kind of hammock at the bottom of your vagina and your clitoris rests on them. They are amazing things. When you're giving birth, assuming it's a normal delivery, when the baby's head comes into contact with the PC muscles, they rotate the head so that it comes out in a twisting motion. Then the shoulders engage with the muscles and these too are twisted. The overall effect is a corkscrew motion, which is better for removing tightly lodged things than the straight-out method, as anyone who's ever opened a bottle of wine can testify. They're great in sex as they give you control over your vagina, allowing you to tighten, relax and pulse it at will. If you strengthen these muscles, you'll also find that your orgasms are more powerful and longer lasting.

- Exercise the PC muscles simply by flexing them – visualize pulling the walls of your vagina together – at every opportunity. You can do this anywhere: at the bus stop, in the car, watching TV, in a meeting. Nobody will ever know – unless you become aroused, which can happen because they make the walls of the vagina contract and produce fluid ready for sex.

- Do sets of ten quick reps when you're starting out with PC exercises, followed by holding the muscles tight for ten seconds. The holding will be difficult at the beginning because your muscles are relatively weak, but before long you'll be working up to twenty-five reps and holding for twenty-five seconds. When you're having a baby, they recommend fifty reps a day – but why not aim for that anyway? You'll soon notice the difference in bed. Remember to breathe, regardless of how much you're concentrating or how aroused you are ...

- Once your muscles have started to develop, you can begin to cater more specifically to sex by inserting a finger and gripping hold of it. Can you feel the difference having worked on it? Now introduce two fingers; now something the size of a penis – like a penis, for example.

A BC Workout

Your man can strengthen his love muscles too. The BC muscles are located below the perineum – behind his penis and just in front of his anus. He can locate them by pulling his penis upwards (no hands) or by visualizing pulling his balls together. As with you, doing this will start to make him ready for sex (in his case, erect), so it's a good exercise if only for those men who've had a long day or are tired, but still fancy a bit. It's best for men *not* to try the exercises at work, however, for obvious reasons.

To train for those mightily powerful orgasms he's about to start having, Candida Royalle, a porn director, recommends that he:

- Gets an erection and then uses his penis to lift a dry flannel.

- Next, he wets the flannel and lifts that.
- Then he should try lifting a dry hand towel; then a wet hand towel.

'Of course, the real winner is the guy who can lift the large wet bath towel,' Royalle says.

No pressure, chaps.

WHAT HAVE YOU LEARNED?

Your man is determined to make you come. What's going to happen in bed tonight?

   a) He'll go down on you for a bit before taking you from behind, which always gets him going.
   b) Having studied this chapter with you and committed a handful of tricks to memory, he'll tell you to relax and enjoy it, then spend literally hours entertaining you with his new-found cunnilingus skills, causing orgasm after orgasm to ripple through you, before gripping your sweat-sheened body in his arms and manoeuvring you into the Ultimo position, which tips you both over the edge.
   c) He'll thrust away as usual in the missionary position ... until you fake an orgasm more or less convincingly.
   d) He'll open this book and follow every sentence step by step, shouting at you when you don't moan in the right places and squinting to read the sex guides as he gives you oral sex, one finger holding his place and the other trying to do something complicated to your G spot.

chapter five
sexual troubleshooting

As we've discovered, sex is a many-splendoured thing. But with it come many not-so-splendid problems, ranging from the psychological to the physiological and beyond. This chapter will help you to tackle some of the most common sexual difficulties. If you can't find what you're looking for, or you're in need of more detailed assistance, please check out my Back Passages (page 155), where you should be able to locate a source of further help.

In the meantime, let's roll up our sleeves and wade into the suspicious and oh so delicate arena of sexual stumbling blocks.

> **DID YOU KNOW?**
> The Chinese and Japanese are the least happy with their sex lives.

UNSEXY AND INACCURATE ASSUMPTIONS

As the director of the FBI memorably put it in *The Silence of the Lambs*: '"To assume" makes an "ass" out of "u" and "me" both.' This book has two whole chapters dedicated to the art of communication, so it's pretty clear how important this is in building a successful sex life with your partner. Making sexual assumptions – about your lover, yourself or even sex itself – leads only to trouble. Talk to your partner instead. Abandon your own inhibitions. Challenge yourself.

Here are a handful of assumptions that may lead to misery, or at the very least concern, on the part of one partner or the other. All of them involve undue expectation of some kind – either of yourself or of your partner – and all of them get in the way of the kick-up-your-heels, carefree sex we should all be working towards. Often, these misunderstandings are hangovers from a time, perhaps fifty years ago, when men and women had very limited and restrictive roles and individuals were not only buttoned up about sex, but had no one to talk to about such subjects. Those must have been very lonely days indeed – thank God the times are a-changin'.

Size Matters

Does size matter? Not really, no. I've only ever been witness to conversations between girls about intimidatingly large penises and what to do when faced with one. Ladies, you probably know all this already. But your partner may not. If he's worried about it (and I doubt he'll tell you directly if he is), subtly reassure him that you devote no time at all to wishing he was bigger. Perhaps leave this book lying around, open to this page, so that he can take in these key *facts*:

- **It's not the mass, it's the motion.** Clichéd, but true.

- **The average penis size is 5.5 inches when erect.** So perhaps not as big as the porn films seem to suggest, then.

- **If anything, it's girth and not length that counts.**
Put in scientific terms, the nerves inside us women can feel its width, but the average vagina is only around 4 inches deep. Although we can cleverly alter our dimensions a little to accommodate a larger man, length means practically nothing to us on the pleasure scale.

> **DID YOU KNOW?**
> In South-East Asia, tribes have been known to implant bells, stones, jewels and shells, among other things, into their penises. These enlarge the penis and are intended to increase the pleasure of the woman. Sometimes they have been fashioned to look like local animals, such as rhinoceroses.

Men Should Initiate Sex

This old-fashioned belief is a surprisingly tenacious little bleeder – and one that must be very wearing indeed for the man in the relationship. If it's always your partner who starts sexual proceedings, how can he ever know for sure that you desire him? If you're a woman who thinks you're not allowed to initiate things, listen to me closely: you're wrong. Set about seducing him. You'll both love it – trust me.

Sex is Only Truly Successful When You Come Together

Blimey, what a load of inferior sex we must all be having most of the time then! And what of taking it in turns to satisfy each other? This is a ridiculous assumption. This kind of climax-centred approach to sex stops couples everywhere having the classy, escapist sex they deserve. Occasionally in your relationship you may have the full Hollywood simultaneous-orgasm shooting match – good for you. But if this is what you're constantly chasing, there doesn't appear to be much potential liberation and relaxation there.

Men are Ever Ready

Nobody is always up for it, and neither partner should take it personally if the other politely declines from time to time. Put a man under too much pressure and 'erectile difficulties', as they call them, are sure to follow. Women: he's not a machine – give your lover a break.

The Older We Get, the Less Attractive Our Partner Finds Us

This is rubbish. Growing old with someone is one of the most amazing things about long-term partnership. If you don't want to listen to me about this, then take it from Tantra. Tantra is a five-thousand-year-old discipline, which sees sexuality as a potential part of spiritual development. It focuses on and embraces the potent sexual energy of women. It isn't a religion; nor an orthodoxy; nor some kind of cult that we either have to join or not. It is more like an approach or an attitude of mind. This means that we can borrow from its teachings and learn from it, without having to commit wholeheartedly to its methods. In other words, we can steal from it freely and not feel guilty.

Tantra focuses on a person's inner soul. Whether or not we choose to focus on Tantra as a discipline, we can all agree with one of its common-sense ideas: that a person isn't simply their age or the way they look. By extension, if we do reduce someone to the way they look, then a long, fulfilling relationship is unlikely to follow.

Despite the impression Western culture might give us to the contrary, men tend to find their partners more attractive as they get older – unless they are chasing a younger model in an attempt to escape from their own ageing process. As tantric writer Val Sampson puts it, 'It may sound brutal, but trying to establish a truly tantric relationship with a man haunted by midlife demons is probably doomed to failure.' Hear, hear to that. She could equally have put 'proper' in place of 'truly tantric'.

Because Tantra is a liberating philosophy, those who take it up often find that it leads to self-acceptance and feeling more sexy in every way. Everyone has met one of those women in their fifties, sixties or seventies who has such an energetic, confident inner glow that she seems effortlessly charismatic and sexy. Now, if you were her partner, would you be searching out a younger model? I rest my case.

TEN COMMON SEXUAL ANXIETIES

1 I Can't Reach Orgasm

You and a huge percentage of Homo sapiens at some time or other. One study found that a quarter of women reported a lack of orgasm in the previous year for several months or more and almost every woman has peaks and troughs in the level of her libido. Worldwide, one in ten men can't get an erection. In other words, a loss of desire in a relationship is entirely normal – as with most things, it's how you tackle the problem when it arrives that counts. And in the vast majority of cases, these difficulties start in the head. If the problems persist, there are organizations and individuals to help you, professionally trained people who will work with you to determine and resolve the root problems. My advice would be to focus your attention on fantasy and masturbation. Exploring your own sexuality – on your own at first, if need be – will enable you to identify what floats your boat, which is a very useful first step.

2 I Can't Come from Penetrative Sex Alone

Most women need clitoral stimulation to be able to orgasm, regardless of the wishful thinking of the world's male population and the impression given in movies, both blue and Hollywood. You and your partner need to master clitoris-friendly positions (see pages 92-99) and while you're about it, he might want to brush up on his cunnilingus techniques too (see page 86).

3 Is Everyone Else Swinging from the Chandeliers the Whole Time?

Of course they're not, silly. On average, most couples reportedly do it twice a week, but everyone has lulls where it happens a lot less than that – who's not affected by being busy at work or hardly getting to see their partner? And as for variety, most of us have three favourite positions that we stick to pretty rigorously. Which doesn't mean this can't change ...

> **Case Study: Carrie**
>
> 'A friend of mine knew a professional couple whom I'd never met, but who were famous with me for not having had sex for a year and a half. Every time I saw my friend, I enquired and every time the answer came: "Still no." Until one day, with a smile, my friend announced, "They have now." What had happened? Just one weekend in Paris without the kids, and they were right back on track. It had a been a very long lull, but they had a strong relationship and that lull eventually came to an end.'

4 My Man Doesn't Like Performing Oral Sex

Many of the sexual problems we have are down to poor communication. You think he doesn't like performing oral sex on you, when in fact he might just be unsure of how to proceed, or had an ex-girlfriend who got 'lonely' when he tried to go down on her – or who teased him about his lack of experience. Get a tongue vibrator (see page 148) and emphasize how brilliantly well they work. Once he's confident at that, tell him how talented he is and make sure he peruses the techniques on pages 86-91.

5 My Partner's More Experienced Than Me

Somebody's got to be. And clocking up sexual partners doesn't equate with being a good lover anyway – far from it. If I had the choice, I'd always go for the partner who'd had a few long-term lovers and learned all the low-down, dirty things that long-term partnership brings. The partner with hundreds of one-night stands to his name suggests to me a partner who's just had hundreds of selfish, drunken fumbles with people he wasn't really in tune with.

6 I Want to Share My Fantasies with My Partner, But I Don't Know How to Begin

Are you opening your mouth to reveal all – but nothing's coming out? Maybe show him the list of women's fantasies on pages 16-17, if you're confident it won't scare him off. Write a sexy letter to him. Or play a game of consequences. Remember that? You begin writing a story, folding over the paper and leaving only the last few words revealed for your partner to add to. Make 'em sexy. Buy erotic fiction, read it and see if his curiosity doesn't get the better of him when you leave the book lying on your bedside table. Rent a female-friendly porn movie and perhaps copy the actors, testing his response. If you're still struggling, create a different persona for yourself and tell him all those things you'd like to do to him through 'her' voice. Those fantasies will soon come tumbling out.

7 My Breasts are Different Sizes

Normal, normal, normal. If your lover has even noticed, he has probably seen something like it before, or he'll think of it as a quirk about you that makes him love you even more. Same goes for if your partner has a kink in his willy. It's normal, but the perceived difference can be exotic. After all, it's not similarity to others that makes a person sexy; it's difference. Difference and attitude.

8 My Jaw Aches When I Give Him a Blow Job

Get good and comfortable at the beginning and don't be afraid to take breaks where you use your hand and/or change your technique – this is all the better for the recipient, too. If he's getting tired going down on you, some techniques for cunnilingus are particularly amenable to pauses or letting you do the work for a while, by moving against his flat, relaxed tongue (see page 89 for more ideas).

9 I Don't Think I'm Very Good in Bed

Well, top marks for caring. Simply lose yourself – in a good way – in his responses to your experiments and you can't go far wrong. The trick to lovemaking is to become totally consumed by the pleasure of giving to someone else. Once you've mastered that – which overrides any confidence problems you might have – the rest follows naturally.

10 I'm Paranoid About My Vagina Smelling Bad

Have you any reason to believe that something's wrong? Have you got thrush? Ask your GP. No? Then you're probably fine. Your smell and taste are individual to you and may vary according to your diet or where you are in your cycle, but any man who's been with others should know that this is simply another aspect of who you are and be into it as a result.

ERECTILE DYSFUNCTION

Impotence is a much more common problem than perhaps you and your partner realize. Help is immediately at hand. If your man's *never* had an erection – primary erectile difficulty – the chances are there's something physically wrong, in which case he should see a doctor. But if it's only *sometimes* that he can't get it up, the chances are he's an average male, perhaps one who's experienced a blow to his sexual confidence in the past.

Because sex is such a singularly touchy subject, women can take a man's lack of erection very personally and react in a defensive way that's quite out of character with our everyday selves. It's obvious, but we should try not to do this. Offering understanding will be received much more positively. A man's impotence has nothing to do with how attractive he finds you – honestly. Yet, in an attempt to retaliate against what we perceive to be the clearest indication possible that he doesn't desire us, we often taunt and reject our lover, which plainly makes the problem worse and persistent.

The 'Give and Get' method, developed by sex therapists Masters and Johnson for men who are experiencing secondary erectile difficulties, puts all this blame and tension in the past. It insists only that as the two of you get down to touching, kissing and stroking (without the act of penetration in sight), that if he gets an erection you stop everything until it goes down, at which point you start again. It may seem counter-intuitive, but it soon teaches him that he can get it up again and again and again, until you are both ready for him to use it. Usually, this works like a charm.

> **DID YOU KNOW?**
> The global average number of times a year that people have sex is 103. The Greeks do it a whopping 138 times a year; the Japanese – the race whose womenfolk are most apt to describe their sex lives as 'monotonous' – have sex an average of only 45 times a year.

INFIDELITY

The dread word. Has it happened to you? It's happened to me and I've never had a feeling like it. I had moved to the other end of the country from the man I was madly in love with, in order to go to college, but even so I sensed something was up, even from that distance, before I'd even spoken to him.

The part of that episode that sticks in my mind is not so much the guessing, or having my suspicions confirmed that my partner had slipped up. No, the real sinking feeling came when I asked him how many times it had happened. I must have known the answer or I wouldn't have so dreaded hearing it. But even so, there was the bottom-dropping-out-of-my-world feeling when the answer came: 'Twice.' As far as I know it never happened again, but I don't know that you can ever be sure after the first time. Let alone when he did it two nights running.

So do you stay or do you go? It's really your call: no one else can make the decision for you. There has to be as good a reason as there can be for you to stay, though. Do you believe him when he says it won't happen again? I guarantee you'll never forget it. Will this cloud the rest of your future together? Can that trust be regained? It's

WEBSITES AND CHAT ROOMS: THE NEW INFIDELITY

So how common is infidelity? In America, 16 per cent of people who are married or living in a committed relationship have cheated on their partner – and nearly twice as many of them are men as women. Thirty per cent of people have fantasized about it. There's also some question these days about exactly what constitutes infidelity. Sounds ridiculous? Well, there's a new kid in town: the Internet.

Perhaps unsurprisingly, men (42 per cent of them) are three times more likely to visit porn sites than women, and 11 per cent of men – 2 per cent of women – have visited sex chat rooms. Men under thirty are by far the most likely demographic to have done both. Perhaps unsurprisingly, again, men are less likely to regard either of these activities as infidelity: 25 per cent of men think that visiting porn websites can be classed as infidelity, as against 42 per cent of women; more men think sex chat rooms constitute infidelity (52 per cent), but a massive 72 per cent of women think visiting a sex chat room is cheating.

Either way, as relationship counsellors will testify, the tensions provoked by these temptations made possible by new technology are beginning to show in relationships. More and more couples are citing them – as well as telephone sex lines – as the final straw that led them to the counsellor's door.

so hard to find any kind of perspective in these circumstances: the temptation is either to dump him or make up excuses for him because you love him. Either way, when push comes to shove, you have to ask yourself if you're ready to move on. All the knowledge, all the advice in the world, means nothing if you're not able to cut your ties with a cheating man.

Of course, the killer fact is that the infidelity may have been symptomatic of a greater problem within the relationship – a problem that you are as responsible for as him. This is what the grown-ups say, and they're right in circumstances where you are withholding emotion or sex, or when both of you don't know who the other is any more.

Yet perhaps you were the guilty party. I grant that there may have been relationship difficulties that drove you to betrayal … but this is never a truly valid excuse, for either of you. Shagging someone else couldn't possibly improve the hostile situation with your partner – so why do it? A moment's pleasure; revenge; perhaps a ducking out of responsibility? After all, if your partner dumps you for infidelity, that's much easier to deal with than the reason being your avoidance of intimacy, say. By far the bravest route is to talk to your partner about any problems – don't just jump into bed with the first guy who comes along. If you're shagging around solely because you want to, face up to this fact and admit it. It's one thing to sleep around if you're single; it's another entirely to cheat on someone for your own selfish pleasure. You can't have your cake and eat it. Have the courage to break up with your boyfriend before you start your sexual experimentation with others.

Tantra on Infidelity

A common attitude towards sex is that once a couple has been together for some time, the spark goes out of their sex life and, naturally enough, either one or both parties are tempted to – and sometimes do – stray to get their kicks.

Case Study: Jenny

'I'm living proof that the consequences of infidelity – of a technological kind – can be fatal to a relationship. My ex, Tom, was not one for spilling his innermost feelings to me, but he was an otherwise enlightened new man. After a number of years of being together, our sex life had begun to ease up. I knew that that was natural, but any attempt I made to discuss it met with stonewalling from Tom. One day, I came back from work early to find him putting the phone down hurriedly. "Oh my God, he's having an affair. I knew it," was my first thought. Tom was mortified and left the room, beetroot red. I dialled to find out the last number ... and it was a premium-rate sex line. Tom had always taken care of the phone bills, but once I got hold of a few previous statements, I realized the extent of his habit. He had spent hundreds of pounds on these lines. Far from going off sex, as I had suspected, he liked to imagine it with some sex kitten conjured up by a hard-up, bored housewife, who was probably doing the ironing while spouting out the same stock of dirty words. Sad to say, the relationship never recovered.'

We think of this as normal, and if a couple manage to avoid it we think they have pulled off some kind of feat. But we are not just animals. Animals are limited and a bit dull in some ways. As far as we know, animals don't have a capacity for reflection or much of an inner or spiritual life.

Tantra encourages people to face the common-sense fact that the sexual energy we experience exists in us, not the other person who suddenly seems to hold all the answers. This stands to reason, whether you like the idea of Tantra or not. It's a version of the idea of taking responsibility for yourself and taking control, rather than

PREMATURE EJACULATION

This is a phenomenon that most of us tend to encounter early on in our sex lives, with randy, over-eager young bucks who can't wait to spill their seed, but it can persist into later life.

Several approaches might help:

- Both of you: use deep breathing when he thinks he's approaching climax, to slow things down and take the emphasis off the act.
- Suggest he works on strengthening his BC muscles (see page 102), just as you'll be strengthening your PC muscles. Then, in bed, he should contract his muscles so that he doesn't reach the point of no return too quickly. The BC muscles surround the prostate, through which semen first has to pass in order to be ejaculated.
- Squeeze his penis — this is a popular choice with sex therapists.

There are also some Taoist- and Tantra-inspired methods, which include scrotal tugging, pressing the perineum and moving sexual energy away from the genitals. For more specialist literature on this subject, perhaps begin with Val Sampson's *Tantra: The Art of Mind-Blowing Sex.*

being some kind of lazy passenger or victim, subject to all the world throws at you and unable to defend yourself against it. So if your sex life is cooling down, don't look elsewhere for that elusive spark. Use the techniques in this book to reignite it yourself.

MORE SHOTS IN THE ARM FOR YOUR SEX LIFE

Whatever the problems disrupting your desire, here are some sure-fire suggestions to kick-start the copulation.

- **Take a detour when you're on a long journey in the car** – and then fuck like bears in a wood. Preferably, choose a wood that doesn't have bears in it, fucking or otherwise. By the time you've found the right wood for your fucking, all that anticipation will ensure that you're both raring to go.

> ### TANTRA ON KEEPING THE SPARK ALIVE
>
> When you're feeling stuck in a rut with your partner, rather than focusing on the quick fix of finding a new person to get you back in touch with your sexuality, Tantra holds that the longer you're with someone, the greater the intimacy and closer the connection and so, potentially, the better the sex.
>
> Day-to-day life – picking children up from nursery, getting stressed at work, hardly seeing your partner – can be the biggest enemy of passion for long-term couples, which makes it all the more crucial to take time with and care of each other.

120 \ while you're down there ...

- **Do a tantric sex workshop together.** You might start off sceptical, but then surprise yourself. And anything that basically worships the force of female sexuality's got to be worth a go, hasn't it?

- **Read a book or smoke a cigarette and challenge your lover to stop you** – using his most finely honed seduction techniques. If you close your eyes or put down the book or the cigarette, he's won and he gets to have his way with you.

- **Go to a swingers' night together.** Resolve just to watch the first time; notice the effect it has on your sex life. If there's a second time, you never know, you may both feel like partaking. If you don't fancy such an immediate time pressure, there are also swingers' holidays. You don't have to do anything, but if the magical chemistry's there, feel free ...

DID YOU KNOW?

Sixteen per cent of women are interested in trying group sex; 26 per cent of men. Less than 1 per cent of women have tried swinging – compared to 5 per cent of men.

- **Get each other hot in the back row of a cinema.** How far can you go without getting thrown out by the management? A good trick: race to the bottom of a family-size carton of popcorn, rip out the bottom and give him a hand job without anyone cottoning on.

- **Go the whole hog in a hotel** – even one in your home town if you have to. Take the lingerie, the essential oils and the porn. Order the champagne and indulge, without having half a mind as to whether you should be doing the washing-up or catching up on that reading for work; without either of you being tempted to answer the phone, resulting in a row.

- **Take photographs of each other naked.** Polaroids have a sexy, spontaneous feel. Or do as sex guru Kate Taylor recommends: take a picture of yourself naked and slip it into his wallet without him knowing – just hope it doesn't fall out when he's handing his business card to an important new client.

- **Join a life-drawing class** (anyway, because they're great) – and then frame and hang the sexiest nude you've created on your bedroom wall. Perhaps pose nude for each other.

- **Acquire a mirror and put it by the bed so that you can watch yourselves at it.** If that's not enough for you, as long as you're not too self-critical to enjoy the fruits of your labour, why not join the ranks of Pamela Anderson and Tommy Lee, as well as Paris Hilton, and make your own blue movie? Just keep your fingers crossed that your partner doesn't post it on the Internet if you split up.

TEXTUAL RELATIONS

If a large proportion of the SMS messages you send each other are not foreplay, then you're misusing the communication medium. Encourage him to plan what he's going to do to you while he's at work and then let you know about it via a saucy text. You do the same for him. And defer gratification – not tonight, but tomorrow.

Did you know?

Americans and Canadians are the most partial to having sex in front of a camera – 21 per cent of them have done it.

WHAT HAVE YOU LEARNED?

You and your man are having sexual difficulties. How do you tackle this problem?

a) Talk to each other about it in an open, blame-free and understanding manner.
b) Have an affair.
c) Start a slanging match.
d) Buy a huge vibrator.

chapter six
spice up your sex life

So, with renewed enthusiasm and vigour, let's get together and rut like Bonobo chimps – who are very naughty indeed. Especially the girls. Here are some secrets for those who want to jazz things up in the bedroom. This chapter is crammed with top tips, erotic extras, suggested sex games and potential practices for a sex life that truly lives up to its promise.

STRIPTEASE

The titillation of the striptease is centuries old and shows no signs of wearing thin. If you think a sexy stripping routine could help rev up your sex life, here are some sure-fire tips to knock your man's socks off. He can always do the same for you, of course.

You will need:

- High heels.
- Attractive undergarments (this is not the moment for those greying granny pants). Perhaps buy yourself a corset, a G-string or a sexy pair of French knickers. Better still, get him to buy them for you.

- Lacy hold-ups. NB: *Not* stockings and suspenders – otherwise you have to cope with the fiddly bit where you undo the catch. Plus, once the stockings are off, you're left with a not-very-erotic flappy belt to deal with. Avoid.
- A feather boa – optional.

Strip Tips

There are two kinds of striptease: the spontaneous walk-through-the-front-door-and-begin-strutting-your-stuff-improvising-with-whatever's-to-hand type (props may include your handbag, car keys, duffle coat, whatever); and the more deliberate variety that involves preparation and a fair degree of thought. A very pampered man is on the receiving end either way. Both styles have their place in a raunchy sex life.

- First, learn to strut a lot – and, specifically, to strut in high heels. No one has ever attempted a striptease without high heels: they're the quickest route to looking like a sex goddess, whatever your stature.

MUSIC TO TAKE YOUR CLOTHES OFF TO

Does he have a favourite tune to which you could strip? Clue: don't use a football anthem. You need to make a decision as to whether you'll use something slow and sensual to seduce him or something with a cracking beat that will demand a funkier routine. One pole dancer I know thinks that Prince's 'Purple Rain' is the perfect song to strip to: in her opinion, it's of just the right length to tease your man and provides atmosphere as well.

spice up your sex life / 125

> ### THE SACRED RULES OF STRIPPING
>
> - No touching by him, however close your arse gets to his face during the course of your routine. Touch him if you like, but I think it's more potent if neither of you make physical contact with each other ... just yet.
> - Keep eye contact with him.
> - Keep touching yourself throughout – make him envy your hands for not being his.
> - Don't hold back. You're stripping for him, for Chrissake – now isn't the time.

- Like most things, stripping is all about attitude. Look like you know what you're doing and he'll never know that you're feeling like a dork inside – he'll be too busy pinching himself, unable to believe what's going on.

- Remove each item of clothing with your back to him and throw the odd coquettish glance over one shoulder. Slow up the more naked you get. This is a tease, remember, not a race to the finish.

- Take the longest time to remove your bra – one strap at a time, perhaps facing away from him again – and make a meal of it by still holding it over your breasts as you turn to face him. Next, put one arm over your breasts and slowly remove the bra from underneath the protecting arm using the other hand, so you remain covered up. Dangle the bra in front of him and drop it into his lap, still without showing him what you've got. When it comes to 'The Reveal' – when you remove your arm – have a really good, involved stroke of your breasts and knead away at

126 \ while you're down there ...

them. I bet he thinks he's going to pass out by now. If he hasn't already.

- Keep strutting around. If you're employing a feather boa or silk scarves in the dance, make like you're using those on your body to get yourself off. Better still, genuinely turn yourself on using them. Caress your whole body: brandish your boa all over your arms, legs, boobs and back and flick it in and out between your thighs.

- Removing your knickers will take practice. Give him a back or side view and ensure that one foot is placed slightly in front of the other. Take it slow. Put your flat palms on either side of your knickers and slowly, slowly lift your knickers away from and down your legs as far as your knees. Keep it leisurely as you step out of them, so as to avoid falling flat on your face.

- Strut some more – trust me, you look amazing.

- After you've finally parted with the high heels that you've become so at home in by now, sit down seductively on a chair.

- Remove your hold-ups by lifting up one leg at a time – giving him a glimpse of his favourite view – then lowering it, so that you can roll each stocking down slowly with the palms of your hands.

- Perhaps finish off your dance by strolling one final time around the room, playing with yourself as you go.

- Now strip him, beginning by undoing his shirt, button by button. Keep the pace teasingly sedate. Finally, let him know when he's allowed to touch you by putting his hands on you.

- Indulge in the hottest sex *ever*.

FANTASIES FOR SHARING

Do you remember back in chapter one when we explored your sexuality and your fantasies? Now might be the time to start sharing some of them with your partner, if you haven't done so already. You might want to go easy on him to begin with, though. Save the more deviant fantasies for when you're ready to get really down and dirty together. He might be alarmed and intimidated by female sexuality unleashed at first, if he's not initiated into it in a responsible fashion.

Turn the tables on him, too. Ask him to tell you all about the first time he climaxed and what he thought about. Hot, hot, hot, this. You'll be playing the role of the naughty eighteen-year-old babysitter in no time, you filthy slut.

> **DID YOU KNOW?**
> Just over half of Americans talk to their partners about their sexual fantasies.

While the fantasies I've urged you to explore on pages 16-17 are more than valid for their unashamed depravity and dense detail, there are more generalized fantasies you can explore with your partner, which are perhaps more suited to being acted out (see page 128). Some of your favourite fantasies may be too intricate, involved or specific for staging in real life – or acting them out might be like seeing a bad film of a beloved novel. Perhaps they're even illegal or too rude to realize. Content yourselves with just describing those ones to each other.

128 \ while you're down there ...

For the adventurous, here are some general scenarios that you might want to bring to life. Remember: this is only an option and not for everyone – but don't knock 'em till you've tried 'em. These suggestions may seem silly to you, a suspension of disbelief too far ... or they may work a treat, releasing your inner animal. Sometimes these things start off with a lot of giggling and an embarrassed 'What are we doing?' – but then proceedings turn suddenly serious, as desire kicks in. Give them a go.

> **DID YOU KNOW?**
> Seventy-one per cent of young adults – aged eighteen to twenty-nine – talk to their partners about fantasies; 55 per cent of thirty- to thirty-nine-year-olds do; 49 per cent of forty- to forty-nine-year-olds discuss fantasies with their lovers.

French Maid

Essentially an excuse for the two of you to use a feather duster to tease each other mercilessly anywhere and everywhere. Feathers on your bottom feel great. Or you could dust each other with icing sugar. A silly persona, yes, but who cares? It's also a chance for him to see you pretending to be servile in a short dress – two things that might not occur on a daily basis.

Professor and Naughty Schoolgirl

A bit more hard core, as there's the possibility of spanking with a hand, whip or cane. On the subject of spanking, concentrate your attention on the area where the buttock meets the thigh for maximum sexual stimulation. And start off with experimental, gentle strokes, obviously. You also need a codeword – perhaps not 'yes' – which you use when things are getting too much. Ditto if you're tying each other up.

Happy Hooker and John

Take this as far as you'd like. He could 'find' you on a street corner when he's 'kerb-crawling'. Then you could do it in the car – away from prying police eyes, obviously. That could spoil things. He might even pay you. I'm sure you wouldn't mind a bit.

Doctors and Nurses

Doctors, make sure you're the ones with the bedside manner, rather than the type who think they're better than the nurses. Nurses, try to be the silly, naughty type rather than the ones with more technical know-how than the doctors and the medical terminology to prove it.

Mrs Robinson and Her Toy Boy

Or, if you lack the imagination/acting skills to improvise this scenario off the cuff, recount your first experiences of masturbation and orgasm to each other. Perhaps you fancied your drama teacher. He's probably still besotted with that older, more experienced babysitter. Where would he have wanted her to touch him? Then where? Like this? Then where? Would he have known what to do then? Would he have done it? Of course he would, the dirty little boy.

firefighter

This one's for your man to act out, obviously. Please suggest he uses grown-up firefighters' gear, rather than something plundered from a kid's toy box, complete with little plastic helmet perched on his head and held on by a thin piece of garrotting elastic. I know he loves to make you laugh, but the comedy routine has to stop at some point so that he can shag you senseless.

Other possible outfits:

For both of you:

- Anything featuring leather, rubber or latex. PVC can look good, but feel awful. And be sensible about what flatters your bodies.

For women:

- Catsuits
- Fishnets
- Hold-ups and high heels (you might want to think about giving him a hand job with a silk stocking while you're at it: he'll love it)
- Corsets

For men:

- Cowboy gear
- Pirate costume – perhaps without the hook and the parrot. Think Captain Jack Sparrow from *Pirates of the Caribbean* instead: sex on sea legs
- Uniforms of most kinds
- Mechanic's overalls – the dirtier the better, or maybe that's just a personal thing ...

Case Study: Jo

'My man and I never thought we'd be into role play. But one night, Andrew went to a school-disco event. You know the kind of thing: everyone dressed up in their old school uniforms dancing to nostalgic hits. Andrew dug out his tie, untucked his shirt and put on some schoolboy shorts. He looked really young, all freshly shaven and adolescent. When he came over to kiss me goodbye, I found to my surprise that I was a bit excited: dampened knickers and a racing pulse. A few weeks later, I suggested to him that he get dressed up again. He was a bit bemused, but I made up some excuse and he obliged. Damn, he looked hot. "You look just like a naughty schoolboy," I said to him. "Are you going to tell me off?" he joked, smiling at me with a definite glint in his eye. "We'll have less of your cheek," I retorted … and then paused. "Actually, we'll have more. Take down your shorts." "I'm sorry?" "Do as I say." "Yes, miss." He was as meek as a lamb – but he still needed to be taught a lesson. Andy bent over with his bum bared, and I beat him firmly with a ruler. "Have you ever been with a woman?" I asked, getting into my stride. "No, miss – but I'd like to, miss," he replied. We were both still laughing a bit self-consciously, but he was obviously getting into it as much as I was by this point. "Well, I'm going to show you what to do. I shouldn't be doing this, of course. We might get caught at any moment. This is totally against the regulations …" Oh my God, the sex was hot – eventually. It was a shock to us both, but this scenario became a regular feature: it was some weeks before Andy finally penetrated "Miss Higgins". We get up to all sorts now, and I can honestly say our sex lives have never been so exciting.'

> ### DRESSING-UP DICE
>
> Once you've got a dressing-up box full of these fantasy outfits, each of you can write down your top three favourites contained therein. Next, number them one to six and throw a dice. Match the number that comes up to the fantasy: one of you then has to dress up for the other and do their bidding.

NB: Realizing our favourite fantasies isn't always the sexual high we hope for, however. Be aware of this potential downside when daring to dabble in the field of fantasy. Both of you should always be completely comfortable with – and excited about – what's going on. The slightest hint of a desire to beat not a bottom but a hasty retreat should be respected by both parties at all times.

Underwear Antics

The attraction of sexy underwear is timeless. A woman in gorgeous undergarments consistently gets guys off. The very act of wearing lovely lingerie is erotic for girls too, of course. When I was in my late teens, I remember trying on a coffee-coloured silk nightie in a changing room. It was one of the most sensual experiences of my entire life, partly because it was completely unexpected. We need to recover that innocent sensuality. And you'll hear no complaints from him.

Although I've suggested a whole host of saucy outfits in the passages above, it's worth us all remembering that dressing up in seductive underwear is just as appealing –

sometimes more so – as doing so in complicated costumes. It's like putting the love back into lovemaking: occasionally, we need to go back to basics to get the most out of our attraction for each other.

You know how sexy you feel if you're wearing alluring undies. Just putting them on can make you feel aroused; at the very least, you're reminded that you're a sexual being, which is never a bad thing. So stock up today. Persuade your man to splash out on you too. After all, he'll be enjoying the benefits at least as much as you will. Let the foreplay commence in the shop for him, as he imagines you in each of the combinations in turn. But make sure he's in the right shop: I doubt you'll go for the trashy red satin number of his dreams. He should start off with tasteful, at least. At the back of this book are some suggested stockists, to point both of you in the right direction (see page 156). One canny lingerie shop owner I know issues little cards to customers that say, 'Mmm – my size at Tallulah is …' for slipping into partners' wallets. Apparently they've worked a treat. If it's too much like hard work to get him to surprise you, go lingerie shopping together. Having said that, in my experience most men will be willing to go that extra mile … especially if it means seeing you gift-wrapped later.

DID YOU KNOW?

Those who wear something sexy are much more likely to see their sex life as great – in other words, where there's effort, there's reward.

Bring Out Your Inner Gimp

DID YOU KNOW?

Eighteen per cent of women and 14 per cent of men describe themselves as 'into bondage'. Sixteen per cent of women and 13 per cent of men describe themselves as being 'into' bedroom spanks.

Fancy a spot of S&M? Sadly, many people do, but never mention it to their partners. Presumably this explains the huge popularity of prostitutes specializing as dominatrixes.

I once went to an erotica exhibition and was browsing a sub/dom stall. For sale were certificates for both parties to sign, which confirmed that their slave/master relationship was consensual. There was a pile of certificates left for women who wanted to be dominated, but the certificates for men had all gone – sold out.

A NOTE ABOUT PIERCINGS

I was once on a hen weekend with ten girls or so, none of whom knew each other at the beginning. To look at them, you'd judge them pretty 'normal'. Then a conversation about piercings cropped up. It turned out half of them had either clitoral or nipple piercings. And they all swore by them. So it's got to be worth a conversation with your partner if you're not too squeamish. As I think everyone knows, for both boys and girls, having someone with a pierced tongue go down on you is supposed to feel wonderful.

You and your partner might not want to take your explorations to such extremes, but consider whether this is a side of sex that might work for you. Be open-minded. Why not use role-play situations to experiment with dominance? What happens if you're the strict schoolmistress and he needs six of the best with your flat, bare hand? And vice versa? A whole new wardrobe and possibly a brand new function for a room in your house may follow.

> **DID YOU KNOW?**
> The French call a quick freshening up of the underarms and genital area a 'tart wash'. Perhaps bear in mind the tart wash when you're too busy being a tart to shower or bathe.

UNUSUAL SEXUAL PRACTICES

If nothing I've mentioned so far is doing it for you, how about one of these more unusual sexual practices?

Coitus à cheval – or coitus on a horse. The motion of the horse is used to aid thrusting.

Flatuphilia. Arousal from having someone pass wind – usually in your face. It happens. I kid you not.

Gerontophilia. Sexual attraction to someone who's significantly older than yourself.

Harpaxophilia. Sexual arousal from being robbed. Mostly this is kept in the realm of fantasy, but have you heard the urban myth of the friend of a friend who did it with someone who was breaking into her house?

Nasophilia. Arousal from the act of seeing, touching, licking or sucking a partner's nose.

Pseudonecrophilia. Sex play where one partner pretends to be dead.

Ochlophilia. Sexual arousal as a result of the presence of a crowd.

Polyiterophilia. The phenomenon of a person being unable to climax without having had several consecutive partners.

Tripsolagnia. Arousal as a result of having your hair played with or shampooed.

Urophilia. Sexual pleasure from acts involving urine.

> ### DID YOU KNOW?
> Icelanders are pretty quirky sexually. When compared to other countries, they have sex the youngest – on average, aged fifteen and a half; they're keener on the idea of free contraception than any other nation (48 per cent support it); and they have the fourth largest average number of sexual partners – at thirteen, the world average is nine – after Turkey, Australia and New Zealand. Maybe it's something to do with all that sunlight for half the year and only darkness the rest.

COMING TOGETHER: THE BRIDGE MANOEUVRE

We've established that the vast majority of women won't come from the thrusting action of penetrative sex alone – unless you use one of those clever positions that also stimulates the clitoris (and both you and your partner are prepared to practise to make the motion, and the angle, perfect). We've explored the fact that simultaneous orgasm is rather rare, and not the be-all and end-all of happy sex.

However, if you must come together once in a while, a trick that every clever girl should keep up her sleeve is the Bridge Manoeuvre. This is when, one way or another, you are taken to the brink of orgasm via clitoral stimulation (whether he is inside you or not at this stage is up to you). Then, with the help of some clever timing, perhaps assisted by a stopwatch and a knowledge of tides, you allow his thrusting (once he is nearly at the point of climax too) to take you both over the edge. A bit of pressure on your clitoris may still be necessary, but since you're most of the way there already, he won't have to make like a jazz drummer on this occasion and do too many different rhythms at once.

SENSATE FOCUS

Sensate Focus is an approach that was first applied to sex around 1970, by sex therapists Virginia Johnson and William Masters. Although originally conceived as a programme to treat impotence, behind it is an ethos that applies to us all: in order to have the best sex, we must change our goal-approached attitude towards it. In essence, the way forward for better bonding and for having the best orgasms is not to chase orgasms.

You may have heard of Sensate Focus without knowing that it had a name. It's simply the practice of taking the emphasis away from anxiety in the head and placing it instead on rediscovering the art of touch. It encourages us to slow everything down. Our whole body is a potential erogenous zone because skin is so incredibly sensitive. It also makes use of that old chestnut delayed gratification, something of which I am a big fan, simply for the oh so stimulating sex that follows the deferral.

A Sensate Focus programme might begin with one half of a couple focusing on touching and the other on being touched, for between fifteen and forty-five minutes. The next day, the toucher and the touched switch roles. The touched may guide the toucher's hand – by touch alone. This carries on for a week. Nothing sexual is allowed. Neither party is allowed to touch the genitals or breasts, or to masturbate. The touching leads nowhere.

There will be nothing directly sexual about the next week either, but more sensual elements might be introduced: a lick or a blow here; the application of a silk scarf or sensual oils there. The couple are encouraged to rediscover the sensual pleasure of kissing again at this point. We forget the effect kissing can have on us – especially when it's all we're allowed!

The third week might introduce masturbation in front of each other at the end of each session; in the fourth week, your man might be allowed to touch your breasts, but nothing else and not until you say he can. Next, you turn your attention to looking at your own body and then that of your partner, telling each other what you like about yourself and each other and describing how you like to be touched.

By the end of this process, fully armed with information about your partner's desires and with your own sensuality reawakened, you are allowed to make love again.

This may seem extreme, but it should be obvious that there are lessons here for all of us. Most of us could learn something and revitalize our sex lives by practising some kind of modified form of Sensate Focus from time to time – if only because slowness, restraint, control and 'not being allowed' are all sexy concepts.

ANAL SEX

There are a couple of myths surrounding this practice, which are perpetuated by both men and women. First, it's not just a thing that men do to women (or to other men). Second, it's not something that women either have to put up with reluctantly to please their man or reject because everyone knows women don't like it. It can be a wonderful experience for a woman – or for a man with a woman and a strap-on, for that matter – but you have to get it absolutely right, and that means slow, slow, slow to start with.

Tips for Back-Door Lovin'

Recipient (for the sake of clarity, you): get relaxed and thoroughly clean at the same time by first going to the toilet and then having a long, languid bath. Maybe bathe with your lover.

Sodomite (your man): loosen the recipient up and relax them even further by making them come once or twice. Make sure your nails are good and short.

Both of you: grease up. This isn't a vagina, so it can't lubricate itself. Help it out with a condom-friendly lubricant (see page 148). Now let's begin.

- Whatever your man does here, he's got to take his time about it. He should start by stroking you generally, and only after that begin kissing and using his tongue on your bum. Suggest to him that he first works away at the area *around* the hole, also massaging and spreading the butt cheeks, rather than forging full steam ahead inside you.

- He might use a small dildo or vibrator to get you loosened up; but don't either of you use the same one inside your vagina that you use in your arse. The same goes for condoms – don't use the same one inside your vagina after this. You could pick up some very nasty illnesses if you do.

- Your partner might want to slip his little finger into your bum at this stage, and then progress slowly upwards in size, until he can insert two fingers. He could maybe use a butt plug to help get you relaxed – and used to the feeling of having something inside you in that intimate place.

- Remind him not to neglect your vagina while he does all this – or the rest of your body, for that matter. The bum appreciates being made to feel like its stimulation is one key part of creating a bigger, whooshy, heady feeling. So your lover shouldn't make it feel like an isolated target: it will ruin everything if he does.

- When it comes to full penetration, your partner could perhaps adopt the method that one male porn star swears by. He sits down, then you lower yourself on to his erection at a rate that you feel comfortable with. But beware: this method might make your butt muscles tense up and actually slow things down. If you prefer, do it doggy style, with him coming at you from behind.

- The first time you try this, perhaps be content with your partner just getting the tip of his (constantly re-lubed) cock in. Feels pretty good, doesn't it? Looks pretty good too, I bet.

- Still, it's not 'Tally ho and away!' just yet. Pause for a moment or two so you can both get used to this feeling … however tempting it is to him to start grinding away like fury.

- At this stage, don't let the fact that *he's actually doing this!* distract your partner's attention from you. Ask him to reach around and stimulate you manually or with a vibrator. Maybe you're happy to do it yourself, but he shouldn't just shut his eyes and revel in living the full porn-star dream. Multitask, man!

- You'll need lots of love afterwards, so please demand this from him. That this act is something of a violation is both part of its appeal and the reason the person being entered should be handled with care throughout. Also, if you orgasm with him inside you in this way, it may be an experience so intense that it's a bit disorientating. I don't know if this is a physiological or a psychological thing, but you may not know what's going on for a moment or two afterwards. Make sure your lover's on hand to help.

Case Study: Ellen

'I've always had a thing about anal sex. It always crops up in my fantasies and is very often the last imagined vision that makes me come. I'd mentioned this desire to my lover, of course, and unsurprisingly he was rather keen. For a long time, all we did was talk about it. Then one day, after we'd been together for about six months, we had a blissful day in Stratford-upon-Avon. It was gorgeously sunny, we took a picnic and several bottles of wine and spent the day lazing on the grass, snacking on strawberries and guzzling chilled vino. When we got back home that night, I was rather inebriated – not falling-all-over-the-place drunk, you understand, just chilled-out, relaxed, letting-my-inhibitions-run-free drunk. I suggested to my partner that we finally go for it. We got into the doggy position and he lined himself up to my bum hole. I was really turned on and really relaxed – so much so that we didn't use any extra lubrication, just a condom, and it didn't hurt me at all. It was an incredible, intense feeling. For a time, we were just immobile, his cock buried deep in my arse and the two of us just taking that in. Then, once I was ready (and had got my breath back), he began to move inside me. It was wonderful. I didn't come, but he did, thrusting inside me and thoroughly enjoying every moment. It's not something we do every time we make love, but we save it for a special, mind-blowing treat every now and again. Oh, and by the way, don't be alarmed or embarrassed if you make a farting noise as he withdraws: it's just natural as both the air and his cock come out of you.'

THE POSSIBILITIES OF PORN

Here are the headlines: these days, not all porn is low-grade, cheaply made, uninspiring, exploitative and for men only. Admittedly, some areas of the industry retain these less appealing qualities. But something of a revolution has taken place. Pornographic material is now available that is not only accessible to women, but damn hot too.

It's a well-known fact that men are visually stimulated when it comes to sex, whereas women are more aroused by the imagination. Think back to those fantasies on pages 16-17: seeing them in glorious technicolour in a hard-core porn movie might well turn you right off. But somehow because you *imagined* what was happening, it was far sexier for you. Though there aren't really hard-and-fast rules about sexual preference – some men will be more moved by imagination; some girls will go for visual erotica; and vice versa – you could summarize this basic difference as:

Men like dirty pictures, girls like dirty books.

Pulsating Fiction

We all know the five or ten dirty words that do it for us. All of these books contain those words in an order that creates sentences.

- 'Mammoth Books of Erotica' (Constable & Robinson).
- Black Lace fiction and 'Confessions'.
- Fantasy books compiled by the author Nancy Friday. There are several available, all highly recommended.
- *Little Birds* and *Delta of Venus* by Anaïs Nin (Penguin Modern Classics).

144 \ while you're down there ...

- *Story of O* by Pauline Réage (Corgi).
- *The Butcher* by Alina Reyes (Vintage).

DID YOU KNOW?
The cleverer you are, the less sex you have.

Sexy Surfing

Thought the Internet was only useful to sexually frustrated male pervs? Well, no: it caters for sexually frustrated female pervs too. And neither of you necessarily needs a credit card to enjoy its fruits. There are a number of erotica websites you can log on to, for instance, which might just float your boat to some sublime sexual destinations. Try www.erotic-readers.com as a starting point.

Girls on Film: One Woman's Journey into Female-Friendly Porn

Porn movies are best known for doing it for men, but they do it for women too. Give yourself a break and try some out – alone at first, if you'd rather.

Before writing this book, my experience of visual porn was limited, although it had begun in my teens. Occasionally, friends would show me copies of their fathers' *Penthouse* that they'd found under the bed, with a mixture of glee and disgust. The pictures were alarming, fascinating, mildly arousing to a teenager. The stories did it for me more, as did the dirty bits of Jackie Collins's books.

As far as 'using' porn went, the only time I can recall was when, some years ago, a boyfriend and I found some abandoned VHS tapes on a London pavement and, intrigued, took them home to see what they were. They were porn. The traditional type: laughably flimsy plot lines, crap music and acting, long-suffering women having it given to them every which way. They were awful, but they did, for a night, ignite a failing relationship.

Then Candida Royalle sent me a handful of her films to look at for this book and a whole new world opened up to me. Royalle was a porn star, who then became a director of porn movies for women, forming a company called Femme Productions. I don't know what I expected from female-friendly porn – butch lesbians? Lots of romance and roses? – but I soon discovered that Royalle knows her audience and all their dirty quirks probably far better than they know them themselves. And her movies work like a dream for men too, since you ask.

Of course, we're not talking *Citizen Kane* with any of these films (and Royalle's are by no means the only female-friendly ones on the market), nor would we expect to be. They are, after all, movies to get off to. But what surprised me is that porn films don't have to be totally functional rubbish. It's like a love affair that's not meant to last, I guess, or like sex itself. Just because something's not profound or forever doesn't mean it shouldn't be carried off with a little flair and panache. And there's something life-affirming about that.

DID YOU KNOW?

Thirty per cent of couples have watched porn movies together.

A HOT MONOGAMY TOY BOX

Last, but by no means least, we come to the topic of toys. Me oh my, but these are incredible things. The sound of a vibrator alone can turn you on if you know what's coming to you. If you're ever having trouble reaching orgasm or feel like your lovemaking's gone a bit lacklustre, these are the babies to banish those blues. If you ever want to learn what your body can do – how many orgasms it might have in a row, for example, or how far you can push yourself – a sex toy is the phone-a-friend you want along for the ride. I cannot recommend them highly enough.

> **DID YOU KNOW?**
> Ninety per cent of us think our sex lives could do with spicing up; 40 per cent think that using sex toys might help.

It's sad to say this after such an impassioned introduction, but ladies, please be warned that sharing your enthusiasm for vibrators with your man can be a chancy business. Men in the army tend to give sex toys to their wives for use while they're away, but on the whole, guys don't encourage a penchant for very sizeable vibrators.

The answer is to involve your man. Show him that this piece of plastic isn't a threat – you still love his cock (and him) a whole lot more. Get your vibe and your man to befriend each other: demonstrate what it can do for him, and what he can do to you with it. It'll be happy families before you know it.

In fact, why don't you and your partner start a collection of sex stuff? Not just vibrators, but cock rings and

> ### Case Study: Maggie
>
> *'When my fiancé bought me a pocket rocket – shiny, modest-sized, designed to fit in my handbag – I was delighted. I was thrilled that he was so open-minded about toys and willing to see that they might help me to reach new heights of sexual pleasure. Then my hen night came along. Inevitably, one of the presents I got was a rabbit vibrator. You know, the Rabbit. Enthusiastically, I showed it to my husband-to-be ... and he went into a sulk for two weeks. I guess he was hurt that I had replaced his pocket-sized effort with something bigger that stimulated me in more ways. Quite literally. Ouch.'*

beads, DVDs and books, blindfolds and special lubricants. You'll have so much fun together, I promise.

Sex Toys: A Rough Guide

There are hundreds and hundreds to choose from: lucky old us. Here are just a select few to entice your interest.

The Rabbit

If you don't have one already (and half the world seems to), do get one of these. The original Vibratex is perhaps the priciest, but still the best. If your partner starts acting like he wants to wring its neck, either acquaint him with the Rabbit or point out it's not real. That sex is more fun with him. (On this occasion, lie if you must.)

Tongue Vibrator

This toy first came to my attention when I was watching Channel 4's *Sex Inspectors*, although it also appeared in *Sex Tips for Girls*. The bloke in the couple featured on the programme was not keen on giving cunnilingus, but the woman was – understandably – keen to receive it. The sex inspectors introduced this vibrator that fitted around his tongue and both of them started really enjoying themselves. The only potential downside is that it will make your man talk funny for a while afterwards, so perhaps then isn't the time to put him under pressure to improve his conversational skills.

You can also get a tongue vibrator for using solo: it's literally a tongue-shaped vibe that performs cunnilingus on you. It looks a little odd, but it does its job very well indeed.

A NOTE ABOUT LUBRICANTS

Sometimes a lubricant will come in handy, whether it's because you're post-menopausal, trying anal sex or at that point in your menstrual cycle when your own juices are not so forthcoming. As a rule, use water-based lubricants such as K-Y Jelly. Oil-based lubricants are harsher on the sensitive microclimate that is your vagina and can also perish latex (i.e. condoms) in less than a minute. Don't use Vaseline down there either – it interferes with the vagina's natural ability to clean itself, which may result in infection.

DID YOU KNOW?

The *Sex and the City* generation – people aged between eighteen and forty-five – are the most accepting of sex toys. The vast majority of them think that the show is responsible for the new-found acceptability of these new-fangled objects.

Nubby G Vibrator

A bestselling G spot vibrator.

Water Dancer

A vibe for the handbag because it is compact and its shape is reasonably discreet. It is also, as the name suggests, waterproof.

Ultime

The favourite of its creator, Candida Royalle, women's porn director supreme, this lovely thing looks like a kind of chic, U-shaped phone. U-shaped so it can stimulate both your clitoris and your G spot. Yum.

Pocket Rocket

This is the beautiful, sleek, shiny, silver vibrator that often appears in illustrated sex books because of the way it looks. If a guy were buying a vibrator for himself, this would be the one he'd choose.

Fukuoko

Dextrous little vibrators that slip on to your fingertips and then get into all sorts of corners with ease. Heaven on your man's perineum; lovely on your nipples.

Hitachi Magic Wand

The great-granddaddy of vibrators – at least in terms of its power. This is a mains-electric vibrator – did you even know there was such a thing? – and tends to be employed by women for whom the stimulation of a battery-operated model is not enough. Which isn't most of us. If you decide to brave it with a vibrator like this, protect your clitoris with a layer of material first or you are in danger of hurting yourself, such is its force!

I Rub My Duckie

A vibrator that looks like a rubber duck. Worth it just for the sheer silliness factor and, frankly, its perv value. Also reaffirms that these are toys and it really is all about fun. And if you choose the travel-size version, you are least likely to suffer embarrassment should your handbag do its upside-down trick.

Crystal Wand

A dildo that can stimulate both a lady's clitoris and her G spot, it's popular because it can be heated up or cooled down before it's used. But I want one mostly because it's such a beautiful thing – with a price tag to match. If I had one, I think I'd get my rocks off just looking at it.

Anal Toys

- Anal beads – for that extra feeling of va va voom, these are designed to be pulled out, one by one, at the point of climax.
- Butt plug – a dildo for your butt.
- Anal vibrator – pretty self-explanatory.

> **DID YOU KNOW?**
> Forty-five per cent of us have bought a sex toy at some time and a further 30 per cent would consider it. Fifteen per cent of people use their sex toys more frequently than they have sex with a partner; 8 per cent of people who possess one have not told their partner about it. Of those who have them, 74 per cent use their sex toys with their partner.

WHAT HAVE YOU LEARNED?

You suggest to your man that the two of you try some new things in bed. He agrees enthusiastically. What happens next?

a) You take a trip to the library and visit the politics section rather than the business section, as is your norm. Both of you pick out a new tome for your bedtime reading.
b) He immediately suggests anal sex and sulks when you say you're not comfortable with the idea. (If only he'd been more patient, you might have come round to trying it.) He refuses to give anything else

a go and says dressing up is 'for girls' when you offer to act out his favourite fantasy.

c) You continue to communicate about the idea via notes on the fridge, both agreeing wholeheartedly that new things in bed are a must, but neither of you commits the time and effort to making that happen. Or to seeing each other in the flesh, for that matter.

d) You browse an online erotica website together, reading some of the porn and turning yourselves on. Daring each other to, you order one of the vibrators on offer. When it arrives, you take it in turns to stimulate each other. It becomes the first toy in a toy box that you add to every month, and marks a new chapter in the ongoing sex life you share together.

conclusion

I do hope that at least some of this info helps. As the old man I mentioned at the beginning of this book made me realize, the sexual journey is a lifelong and potentially lonely one. 'Lifelong' in that we never stop learning – because, hopefully, we don't stop having sex. 'Lonely' in that we don't always talk about sex that much.

This may be obvious, but talking and clarifying is a habit like any other. A strange thing happened to my partner and me during the writing of this book: we became pathological clarifiers and explainers of what we were saying to each other. It all started when I was writing about men and women generally. Just as when you get new shoes you notice everybody else's, I began to see evidence of men and women's fundamental differences everywhere and on a daily basis. I thought it was so interesting that I told my partner about it. Then he, too, began to see it, both in our relationship and in those of others. It's everywhere; it's nobody's fault; and in fact it's brilliant. Keep the communication channels open and these differences needn't be a destructive force – they'll be an aphrodisiac instead.

One last thing has occurred to me. If you ever think you should be on your own or that you're with the wrong person, of course you may be right. You may be right … or the alternative scenarios which you conjure up in your mind might in reality be as fantastical, and ultimately unfulfilling, as having sex with an entire rugby team or any of the other filthy things that women think up in their spare time to get off.

It's an old-fashioned view, and if you're genuinely unhappy, an unhelpful one, but being in a relationship that has managed to endure does have some value in itself. As for sex, it's the foundation for the dirtiest kind of all. Go on, start talking to each other. Reassure each other that you're safe – and then take off into uncharted sexual territory. Together you can come up with adventures more risqué than even your wildest dreams have made. Start today. Play.

THE FIRST SECRET OF SUCCESSFUL SEX

TURN OFF THE TV AND GET TO IT!

appendix
back passages

HELP IS AT HAND

Sexual Health and Family Planning

- www.brook.org.uk – advice, counselling and medical help on contraception, pregnancy, abortion and sexual health.
- www.fpa.org.uk – family-planning association for improving the level of education and sexual health in the UK.
- www.impotence.org.uk – a harshly named organization dealing with all sorts of problems in male and female potency. As my partner put it, 'They might as well call it floppy.com.'
- www.netdoctor.co.uk – for information on all aspects of health, including sexual health.
- www.nhsdirect.nhs.uk – for help on all health issues, including information about local clinics for those with STDs and those who need family-planning services.
- www.plannedparenthood.org – for support and information on birth-control issues in the US.
- www.womenshealthlondon.org.uk – for information on all aspects of women's bits and how they work.

Counselling

- www.rapecrisis.co.uk – referral services for women who have been raped or sexually abused.

- www.relate.org.uk – provides education, support and counselling for couples and families.
- www.survivorsuk.org – for men who have been raped or sexually abused.

SUGGESTED STOCKISTS

Erotic Extras

- www.annsummers.com – lingerie, DVDs, toys. Recently revamped and now present on the high streets of most major towns in the UK, as well as online. Ann Summers parties can be great fun, too. Why not look into hosting one for you and your girlfriends?
- www.coco-de-mer.co.uk – a very high-class 'erotic emporium' in London and online, containing all sorts of weird and wonderful merchandise for the discerning consumer of the erotic. Carefully designed to appeal to women and couples, as well as men. It also offers experts in all aspects of the erotic arts, who are willing to teach you what they know – either in the boutique or in the comfort of your own home.
- www.lovehoney.co.uk – sex toys and erotic literature online.
- www.sh-womenstore.com – another gorgeous erotic emporium in London (and online) this time catering specifically for women.

Underwear

- www.agentprovocateur.com – truly sumptuous underwear … but if you're a big-breasted lady and you don't want to end your shopping expedition in tears, forget it.
- www.bravissimo.com – thank you, thank you, thank you. Bras and underwear for curvy ladies that actually don't look like scaffolding. Available via catalogue, and at more and more stores across the UK.
- www.rigbyandpeller.com – classy, sometimes lovely underwear

by appointment to Her Majesty the Queen. Corsetieres to the Queen since 1960 and able to accommodate the larger lady. Buy online or at one of their London stores.
- Tallulah Lingerie, 65 Cross Street, London N1 2BB – no website, but well worth a visit.
- www.victoriassecret.com – gorgeous underwear for the American lady and the online shopper, for those of a 'full-figure DD' size or below.

NICHE SITES, EVENTS AND COURSES FOR THE CURIOUS

- www.diamondlighttantra.com – for UK-based Tantra workshops.
- www.fyeo.co.uk – pole- and table-dancing lessons in a gentleman's club in Mayfair, London – in case you get a taste for it after the stripping tips contained in this book.
- www.londonfetishfair.co.uk – home of information on the London Fetish Fair, which is held monthly, providing you with the opportunity to purchase a vast array of merchandise, including 'bondage systems'.
- www.nightofthesenses.com – an annual event for charity with all kinds of weird and wonderful aspects to it: fantasy fayre, lesbian lounge, lap dancing for couples and silhouette frottage.
- www.sexsecretsrevealed.com – for tips on all the fun bits of doing it and how to make them even better.
- www.swingeradz.com – online personal ads for swinging couples. You don't have to reply; you could just look together and imagine ...
- www.tantra.org – for Americans interested in Tantra.
- www.vday.org – for news of the work of Eve Ensler (of *The Vagina Monologues* fame) and others to stop violence against women and girls.

bibliography

Chia, Mantak, with Dr Rachel Carlton Abrams, *The Multi-Orgasmic Woman: Sexual Secrets Every Woman Should Know* (Rodale International Ltd, 2005)

Cox, Tracey, *Supersex* (Dorling Kindersley, 2002)

Dickens, E., *This Book Will Get You Laid* (Michael O'Mara Books, 2006)

Ensler, Eve, *The Vagina Monologues* (Virago, 2001)

Evans, Dylan, *Emotion: The Science of Sentiment* (Oxford University Press, 2001)

Godson, Suzi, with Mel Agace, *The Sex Book* (Cassell Illustrated, 2002)

Goleman, Daniel, *Emotional Intelligence: Why It Can Matter More Than IQ* (Bloomsbury, 1996)

Kerner, Ian, *She Comes First: The Thinking Man's Guide to Pleasuring a Woman* (Souvenir Press, 2005)

Love, Brenda, *Encyclopedia of Unusual Sex Practices* (Greenwich Editions, 1999)

Miller, Geoffrey, *The Mating Mind: How Sexual Choice Shaped the Evolution of Human Nature* (William Heinemann, 2000)

Pease, Allan and Barbara, *Why Men Don't Listen and Women Can't Read Maps* (Orion, 2001)

Pease, Allan and Barbara, *How Compatible Are You?* (Orion, 2005)

Quilliam, Susan, *Staying Together: From Crisis to Deeper Commitment* (Vermillion for Relate, 2001)

Ridley, Matt, *The Red Queen: Sex and the Evolution of Human Nature* (Penguin Books, 1993)

Royalle, Candida, *How to Tell a Naked Man What to Do* (Piatkus Books Ltd, 2005)

Sampson, Val, *Tantra: The Art of Mind-Blowing Sex* (Vermillion, 2002)

Sonntag, Linda, *Great Sex Techniques* (Hamlyn, 2002)

Sussman, Lisa, *Over 100 Triple-X Sex Tricks* (Carlton Books for *Cosmopolitan*, 2005)

Taylor, Kate, *A Woman's Guide to Sex* (Hamlyn, 2004)

index

anal sex 23, 139-42, 151

clitoris 23, 27-8, 109, 149, 150
   sexual positions for stimulation of 92-9, 137
communication 35-59
   exercises for improving 46-9, 60-2
   how-to guides to 43-6, 49-51
cunnilingus 84-91, 109, 112, 148
   how-to guide to 86-91

erogenous zones 21, 78-84, 138

fantasies 15-8, 57, 74, 111, 142, 143
   for sharing 127-32
   women's 16-7

G spot 28-30, 97, 149, 150

impotence 109, 113
infidelity 114-9

kegel muscles 22, 100-3, 118
kissing 82, 83, 138

lubricant 140, 147, 148

massage 67-8, 79
masturbation 18-9, 20, 25, 32, 63, 109, 129, 138
   importance of 12-5, 24
   mutual 70-1
   tips on 24-6

pornography 17, 74, 111, 120, 143-5
   books 143
   films 144-5
   websites 115, 144
pregnant sex 74-5
premature ejaculation 118

relationship 37-8
   reigniting your sexual 60-2, 65-71, 119-21, 123-51
   tips on improving your 43-6, 46-9, 50, 57-9
role play 127-32, 135

sadomasochism 18, 72, 134-5
Sensate Focus 137-9
sex 12-34, 50, 56-75, 77-103, 123-51
   anxieties about 108-14
   assumptions about 31, 45, 104-8
   men and 62-4
   myths 71-5
   positions 74, 92-9, 137
   science of 37, 61, 63, 106
   unusual practices 135-6
sex toys 23, 25, 27, 74, 80, 110, 140, 141, 146-51
striptease 123-6

Tantra 82, 107-8, 116-9, 120

vagina 19, 20, 21-2, 24, 26, 29, 89, 91, 101, 106, 112, 140, 148
vibrators *see* sex toys